'In this groundbreaking work, Orna Afek offers a fresh and insightful perspective on psychoanalysis, examining its development through the lens of narcissism. With remarkable clarity and depth, Afek exposes a critical gap in mainstream psychoanalytic theory: the undervaluation of interpersonal relationships as a fundamental human need. By exploring the narcissistic traits of influential theorists and their impact on psychoanalytic thought, Afek presents a compelling case for a more balanced approach. This book is an essential read for clinicians, researchers, and anyone interested in the evolution of psychoanalysis. Afek's work not only challenges established paradigms but also paves the way for a more holistic understanding of the human psyche.'

Prof. Aner Govrin, *Editor of* Routledge Introductions to Contemporary Psychoanalysis, *Director of the doctoral program "Psychoanalysis and Hermeneutics," Bar Ilan University, Israel*

Psychoanalysis Through the Lens of Narcissism

This critical historical review of psychoanalytic theory and practice reflects on the place of psychoanalysis in contemporary Western culture in light of its preoccupation with the self and associated failure to emphasize the role of close interpersonal relationships as central to the human psyche.

The elusive presence of the separate other in psychoanalytic theory is discussed vis-à-vis the life stories of Freud, Winnicott, and Kohut. The underlying narcissistic bias in the theories of these three pioneers of psychoanalysis – classical Freudian drive theory, Winnicott's theory of the parent-infant relationship, and Kohut's theory of self-psychology – is traced back to their narcissistic personality traits, which impacted their views and perceptions and obscured the fundamental centrality of interpersonal relationships per se in the inner world of the individual, with far-reaching implications for psychoanalytic thought and practice.

With fresh insights on the subjectivity of personality theories, the core features of the narcissistic personality, and the implications of the narcissistic position for theory and clinical practice, this book will interest psychotherapists, psychoanalysts, and other professionals in the field, specifically those interested in personality diagnosis, narcissism, attachment theory, and psychotherapeutic approaches and psychoanalytic theories in general.

Orna Afek, MA, is a senior clinical psychologist and head of the Tamuz Institute for Psychotherapy, established by her in 1994. She also serves as a supervisor and lectures on critical evaluation of psychoanalytic theories, narcissism, dream analysis in psychotherapy, and personality diagnosis, which are her main areas of interest.

Evolutions in Psychoanalysis Book Series
Daniel Goldin and Melvin Bronstein
Series Editors

Under the editorship of Melvin Bronstein and Daniel Goldin, the Evolutions in Psychoanalysis book series provides a shared space for writers who are eager to revisit formative psychoanalytical ideas in often innovative new ways. The word 'evolve' literally means 'to unroll', and the contemporary use of the latter term suggests that something new can be revealed through a process of incremental unravelling. As a definition of both the aspirations of this series and of psychoanalysis itself, this understanding exemplifies the possibility that one can take apart by creating and create by taking apart.

The volumes in this series do not represent a particular school of psychoanalytic thought, but rather comprise and encourage new voices from all schools and spaces – across time and geographical location – in the knowledge that brilliant thinkers and ideas can emerge from unforeseen places. The series does also encompass the editors' interests in how contemporary psychoanalysis intersects with society and culture at large; differing analyses of the micro-processes that take place in clinical encounters; and the influence of other disciplines – such as philosophy and infant-research – upon the field of psychoanalysis, and welcomes contributions to these and other topics.

Of critical importance to the formation of this series is its aspiration to foreground voices from marginalized ethnic groups, for the vitality and creativity they offer which is so necessary to the field, and to continue in the direction of redress and repair for the omissions and exclusions of the past.

For more information about this series, please visit: https://www.routledge.com/Evolutions-in-Psychoanalysis-Book-Series/book-series/EVIPS

The Storying Mind
Bringing Nature, Nurture and Culture Together in Psychotherapy and Everyday Life
Daniel Goldin

Rediscovering Sandor Ferenczi
Arnold Wm. Rachman's Contribution to the Sandor Ferenczi Renaissance
Kooden and Larriviere

Psychoanalysis Through the Lens of Narcissism
Orna Afek

Psychoanalysis Through the Lens of Narcissism

Orna Afek

Translated by Hanni Manor

Routledge
Taylor & Francis Group
LONDON AND NEW YORK

Designed cover image: A man touching his reflection in the water – stock illustration. Cargo/Imagezoo via Getty Images.

First published 2025
by Routledge
4 Park Square, Milton Park, Abingdon, Oxon OX14 4RN

and by Routledge
605 Third Avenue, New York, NY 10158

Routledge is an imprint of the Taylor & Francis Group, an informa business

Translated by Hanni Manor

British Library Cataloguing-in-Publication Data
A catalogue record for this book is available from the British Library

Library of Congress Cataloging-in-Publication Data
Names: Afek, Orna, 1959– author.
Title: Psychoanalysis through the lens of narcissism / Orna Afek ; translated by Hanni Manor.
Description: Abingdon, Oxon ; New York, NY : Routledge, 2025. | Series: Evolutions in psychoanalysis book series | Includes bibliographical references and index.
Identifiers: LCCN 2024042127 (print) | LCCN 2024042128 (ebook) | ISBN 9781032885322 (hardback) | ISBN 9781032884332 (paperback) | ISBN 9781003538295 (ebook) | ISBN 9781040300282 (adobe pdf) | ISBN 9781040300299 (epub)
Subjects: LCSH: Narcissism. | Psychoanalysis.
Classification: LCC BF575.N35 A34 2025 (print) | LCC BF575.N35 (ebook) | DDC 150.19/5—dc23/eng/20241104
LC record available at https://lccn.loc.gov/2024042127
LC ebook record available at https://lccn.loc.gov/2024042128

ISBN: 978-1-032-88532-2 (hbk)
ISBN: 978-1-032-88433-2 (pbk)
ISBN: 978-1-003-53829-5 (ebk)

DOI: 10.4324/9781003538295

Typeset in Optima
by Apex CoVantage, LLC

For my sisters and brothers, who share in the innermost layers of my soul

Contents

About the author

Ms. Orna Afek, MA, is a senior clinical psychologist with a track record of over 30 years in psychotherapy and psychodiagnosis. She heads the Tamuz Institute for Psychotherapy (https://www.mtamuz.com/en), established by her in 1994.

With branches across Israel, Tamuz Institute offers a range of psychodynamically oriented psychotherapy and counseling services as well as guidance and training courses for clinical psychology interns on various psychotherapeutic approaches and psychodiagnostic methods, conducted for the most part by Ms. Afek.

Ms. Afek also serves as a lecturer at the School of Jungian Analytical Psychotherapy of the Kibbutzim College of Education, Technology, and the Arts in Tel Aviv and conducts continuing education programs for professionals in various forums.

Topics covered in the various courses offered include:

- Comprehensive personality diagnosis (according to the PDM-2)
- The use of dream analysis in psychotherapy
- Comparative evaluation of psychoanalytic theories
- Understanding the narcissistic personality – diagnosis and therapeutic implications

Seeking to share the insights she obtained as a clinical psychologist and supervisor with colleagues in the psychoanalytic community, Ms. Afek has authored scholarly papers on these and other issues, in both Hebrew and English, published on the websites of Tamuz Institute and Hebrew Psychology, the community of mental health professionals in Israel.

Two papers by Ms. Afek published in *Psychoanalytic Psychology* (https://doi.org/10.1037/pap0000161; https://doi.org/10.1037/pap0000201) deal with narcissism, her specific field of interest, on which she further elaborates in this book.

Ms. Afek holds a BA in Psychology (1984) and an MA in Clinical Psychology (1987), both from Bar-Ilan University, Israel.

Preface

Psychoanalysis has undergone substantial changes in the course of its development since Freud laid the foundation for understanding human psychology. While the body of psychoanalytic knowledge offers invaluable insights into the complexities of the human psyche, it is argued that there is a major lacuna in mainstream psychoanalysis, namely, its failure to take due account of the significance of interpersonal relationships per se as an inborn fundamental need, irrespective of any function they may serve (e.g., mirroring, containment, fulfillment of physical needs, providing emotional security, or fostering self-worth), as discussed at length in Chapter 1. We humans are tied to each other in various ways, we need each other's company, we are emotionally and mentally engaged in our interpersonal relationships, and we are bound together by an affective bond and attachment relationships that are central to the human psyche. Yet the feelings of longing for a loved one, the close emotional relationships between siblings or friends (beyond the natural attachment between children and parents), the void left by a departed significant other that no one can fill, and the deep-seated need for social involvement and interaction with others – all these were largely overlooked for decades by psychoanalysis while its focus was on the self.

Preoccupation with the self and its needs to the virtual exclusion of the other and disregard of the significance of the other in the life of the individual are key characteristics of narcissism. The phenomenon of narcissism is enlarged on in Chapter 3, and three core features of the narcissistic personality are suggested – grandiosity, schizoidism, and the difficulty acknowledging the otherness and separateness of the other. As far as the narcissist is concerned, the other is there to serve him and fulfill his needs as a mere background actor in the self-scripted drama taking place in his inner world. When displayed by a theorist, the narcissistic self-centeredness is bound to be reflected in his theory, specifically a theory that deals with the human psyche, since the personality and subjective world of the theorist inevitably color his thinking, as demonstrated by psychobiographical analysis. The inevitable subjectivity of personality theories, in general, and psychoanalytic theory, in particular, is discussed in Chapter 2, and the need for analyzing and understanding the subjective world of the theorist and its impact on his theory is highlighted. In this context, Strozier (2001) is cited as noting, "Perhaps any thinker, especially a psychological one, draws on his or her own conflicts as the basis of insight. The question, however, is not whether theories are subjective but whether such insight can be generalized" (p. 260).

Based on the psychobiographical literature on Freud, Winnicott, and Kohut as well as on their writings, the narcissistic personality traits shared by these three pioneers of psychoanalysis as reflected in their lives and, even more important, in their theorizing are discussed in depth in Chapter 4 with reference to the three core features of narcissism suggested in Chapter 3. As shown, their narcissistic personality traits colored their views and perceptions and blinded them to the fundamental centrality of interpersonal relationships in the inner world of the individual.

At the same time, other theorists in the psychoanalytic school highlighted the essential role of interpersonal relationships in the organization of the human psyche, challenging the then dominant, narcissistically biased Freudian drive theory and its emphasis on the primacy of instinctual drives in human psychology. However, for years, their theories were dismissed, and they were pushed to the margins by the psychoanalytic establishment. Chapter 5 discusses the significant contribution of four prominent theorists marginalized due to their groundbreaking views – Ferenczi, Balint, Fairbairn, and Bowlby – who had a far-reaching impact on psychoanalytic thought, shifting its focus toward relational and intersubjective perspectives.

The relational intersubjective school has gained momentum in recent decades and brought into the mainstream the once marginalized theorists. Yet while the narcissistic bias in psychoanalytic theory has been thus attenuated, it is still reflected in the relational intersubjective approach and its clinical practices as demonstrated, inter alia, in the excessive focus of relational and intersubjective theorists and practitioners on the development of the self and associated failure to address real-life interpersonal relationships, as discussed in Chapter 6.

The shift of trend toward relational and intersubjective perspectives is not limited to any specific psychoanalytic school, but rather is taking place across the field, as evidenced, for instance, in recent psychoanalytic views on loss and grief processes, which are discussed in Chapter 7. This significant and, in my view, welcome change of trend in psychoanalytic theory and practice shifts the focus toward the fundamental centrality of interpersonal relationships per se and their essential role – over and beyond sustaining the self – in the organization of the human psyche and the psychic life of the individual.

Finally, I reflect in Chapter 8 on the current status of psychoanalysis as a therapeutic method and its apparent failure in many cases to take due account of the patient's life reality and answer his specific needs. An alternative non-narcissistic, in-depth psychotherapy is proposed in conclusion that responds to the patient's specific needs while considering the broad picture of his personality and life reality.

Note: For the sake of simplicity, the masculine form is used throughout this book to refer to both men and women.

Reference

Strozier, C. B. (2001). *Heinz Kohut: The making of a psychoanalyst*. Farrar, Straus, and Giroux.

Acknowledgments

I would like to express my deepest gratitude to Hanni Manor ((https://words ofhanni.com/) for her inspired translation of my manuscript from Hebrew into English. Her in-depth understanding of academic writing, creative approach, attention to detail, and dedication to the task have significantly contributed to my work.

Orna Afek

1 The elusive presence of the separate other in psychoanalytic theory and practice

Relatedness versus self-definition

Blatt (2008) described two fundamental dimensions of the human experience – relatedness and self-definition – that when kept in balance enable healthy functioning of the personality. The dimension of self-definition (introjective dimension) concerns cognitive and emotional focus on issues of self-identity, self-worth, the need for recognition, the endeavor to achieve personal goals, the fear of loss of control, the striving for autonomy, and so on. The dimension of relatedness (anaclitic dimension) concerns issues of dependence on the other, abandonment anxiety, intimacy, empathy and care for the other, reciprocity and cooperation in interpersonal relationships, and so forth. According to Blatt, personality development involves an ongoing effort throughout life to achieve a balance between interpersonal relatedness and self-definition, and when the balance between these two polarities of experience is severely disrupted, psychopathology emerges. Thus, narcissistic personality disorder reflects an exaggerated and distorted emphasis on the dimension of self-definition. The narcissist is preoccupied with himself and his self-worth and has no interest in others or in relationships with others, except as regards any function they may fulfill for him. The paranoids are also classified in the self-definitional domain. While the latter are preoccupied, in a sense, with the other, their apparent interest in the other is driven by suspicion, anxiety, and hostility and actually serves as a defense against the other, whom they perceive as threatening and from whom they seek to distance themselves. The obsessive-compulsives, who are also classified as self-definitional, are primarily concerned with accomplishing tasks and achieving goals while the other and relationships with the other are seen by them as unworthy of their time and energy. In contrast, the dependent, borderline, and histrionic personality disorders reflect a drastic shift toward the dimension of interpersonal relatedness. Dependent individuals seek the support, advice, and guidance of others and tend to trust and rely on others rather than on their own judgement. Borderline individuals are preoccupied with measuring their emotional closeness to or distance from others, while the real or imagined threat of abandonment casts a dark shadow over their

DOI: 10.4324/9781003538295-1

lives. The histrionics are dependent on the love of others, and seeking to feel loved and desired, they are constantly engaged in alluring others. The distinction made by Blatt between these two fundamental dimensions or polarities of the human experience is in line with the dialectics of autonomy and mutuality discussed by other theorists. Bakan (1966), for instance, suggested the concepts of agency and communion as the opposite poles embodying the duality of human existence, where agency manifests itself in self-preservation, self-assertion, and self-development, while communion is displayed in extroversion, openness, and sociability.

Blatt (2008) presented a comprehensive and fascinating historical review, illuminating the place given to the domains of relatedness and self-definition in different cultures through the centuries. As noted by Blatt, individualism is a relatively modern concept in Western culture. While it has its roots in ancient Greece and Rome, it was only in the late 13th century that it reemerged in Europe. Thus, in the preceding centuries of the Middle Ages, when individuality and personal freedom were suppressed, the arts of portrait painting and autobiographical writing were rarely practiced, and artists seldom signed their works of art. The emergence of individualism was a significant milestone as it set in motion momentous processes related to human rights and personal well-being, autonomy and self-realization, scientific and technological development, and more. Persons who cultivate their individuality are autonomous and independent, have initiative and free will, are aware of their needs and wishes, and can realize their full potential – qualities that inspire deep feelings of satisfaction, enjoyment, and self-worth and may be channeled to the benefit of society. However, the other side of the self-definitional coin is manifested in narcissistic preoccupation with the self at the expense of enjoyable mutual interpersonal relationships, which are an important aspect of the human experience that has been pushed aside in contemporary Western culture. Yet, as noted, both self-definition and relatedness are fundamental dimensions of the human experience and hence have to be considered in any theory of human psychology.

In this context, a distinction should be made between merely functional, utilitarian interpersonal relationships, which are solely designed to serve the self and should thus be categorized under the self-definitional domain, and interpersonal relationships per se, maintained apart from and irrespective of any need they may fulfill, which, as shown hereinafter, have an essential role in the inner world of the individual. We humans have an inherent, deep-seated need to relate to and connect with others; we enjoy social interaction and collaboration with others; we care for others and show empathy and consideration for others even when it goes against our own narrow interests. A range of theories and studies cited by Blatt (2008) provide support for the relational view of human nature and demonstrate that we are tied to each other in various ways and that interpersonal relationships are fundamental to our existence. Noteworthy in this context is Blatt's reference to Darwin's theory of evolution and natural selection, which advocates the principle of survival of the fittest. As noted by Blatt, recent developments in evolutionary biology show that communality, altruism, and cooperative rather than egocentric behavior create an evolutionary advantage in the struggle for survival. Examples of prosocial behavior displayed by various species, including but not only humans, demonstrate, according to Blatt, that mutual commitment is biologically innate and not necessarily contingent on education or culture. Thus, in one of the studies referenced by Blatt, field researchers have observed empathetic behavior among unrelated vampire bats that shared food with starving cave mates. Along the same lines, Mitchell (2000/2023), one of the prominent advocates of the relational perspective in psychoanalysis, discussed the prosocial behavior displayed in nature:

> In what sense does a bee seek other bees? In what sense does the wolf or zebra seek other members of his pack or herd? It seems cumbersome and improbable to regard this gregariousness or object-seeking as expressive of a discretely experienced need, like hunger or sex, that emerges from time to time, when the individual bee or wolf or zebra feels lonely, requiring other members of its kind for satisfaction. Many animals are, by their very nature, social beings and can exist as a normal creature of their specific type only as part of the group.
>
> (p. 105)

Bowles (2006) traced the evolution of human altruism to early human groups, showing how group solidarity and cooperation between fellow group members supported and were essential to their survival.

As argued, interpersonal relatedness is fundamental to human existence. Indeed, it goes far deeper than mere functional relationships or casual social ties. The basic human need for a close intimate relationship and emotional attachment to a significant other regardless of and apart from the fulfillment of needs is exemplified in the relationship between parents and children. Naturally, children need their parents as protective and caring figures who provide food; teach, reassure, and calm them; mirror and enhance their self-image; acknowledge their individuality and personal autonomy; and so on. However, important as these functions are, they cannot replace the unique emotional attachment between parent and child. No substitute parental figure, loving as that figure may be, can heal the wounds or fill the void left by an absent parent, whether the child has been abandoned or the parent disappeared under any other circumstances. This was aptly illustrated by Fairbairn. As related by Mitchell and Black (1995/2016), Fairbairn wondered, reflecting on his clinical work with children who were living with an abusive parent, how it could be that the abused child was still clinging to the abusive parent despite the pain:

> He decided it was one's *lived experience* growing up, not the expression of internally arising drives, that was shaping the lens through which we

> organize and understand our experience with others. Fundamentally people are searching for connection, not for drive satisfaction. It is this deep yearning that leaves us so vulnerable to the impact of our earliest experience. That particular experience, he concluded, becomes the model, the internalized organizing template, defining for each of us what it means to love another person.
>
> (p. 379)

As Mitchell (2000/2023) further noted, "Fairbairn was suggesting that object-seeking, in its most radical form, is not the vehicle for the satisfaction of a specific need, but is the expression of our very nature, the form through which we become specifically *human* beings" (p. 105). It is thus the fundamental human search for relatedness rather than for drive satisfaction, as argued by Freud, and specifically the innate need for close intimate relationships and emotional attachment, irrespective of the fulfillment of needs, that play an essential role in personal development and individual psychodynamics.

The underlying narcissistic bias in psychoanalytic theory and practice

While psychoanalytic theory has undergone substantial changes in the course of its development since Freud laid the foundation for understanding human psychology, its underlying narcissistic bias has been reflected over the decades in its focus on the self and associated failure to place due emphasis on the essential role of interpersonal relationships per se as central to the human psyche. As argued and shown in the following chapters, by and large, psychoanalysis failed to address the innate need for interpersonal involvement and social interaction, the natural empathy for the other and enjoyment in sharing with others, and the inherent quest for emotional attachment to a significant other. It should be noted, though, that theorists such as Ferenczi, Balint, Fairbairn, and Bowlby, who highlighted the fundamental significance of parent-child attachment in psychological development, as well as others known as the neo-Freudians, among them Sullivan, Horney, Fromm, and Thompson, who emphasized the role of social and cultural factors in shaping personality, laid the groundwork for reorienting psychoanalytic thought and shifting its focus toward relational and intersubjective perspectives. Alas, at the time, those architects of the relational model were pushed to the margins, and it is only in the last decades that they were brought into the mainstream by theorists associated with the intersubjective relational approach – Mitchell, Benjamin, Aron, and Stolorow, among others. The theories of Ferenczi, Balint, Fairbairn, and Bowlby and the valuable contribution of the relational model they offered toward understanding the mental world of the individual are discussed at length in Chapter 5. Chapter 6 is centered on the intersubjective relational approach, which has gained momentum in the psychoanalytic community, in particular, in the United States. Its significant contribution to the paradigm shift in contemporary psychoanalysis is discussed in that context and, at the same time, the spotlight is turned on the underlying narcissistic bias that is still reflected in the intersubjective relational approach and its clinical practices.

It may then be argued that psychoanalytic theory – "even in its relational versions," as Rubin (1998, p. 134) put it – has contributed its share to the predominant self-centered position of contemporary Western society. As Blatt (2008) noted, "Psychological theories have traditionally given much greater importance to the development of individuality or self-definition than to interpersonal relatedness as the primary feature of the mature individual" (p. 16). In the same spirit, Rubin (1998) discussed the failure of psychoanalysis to consider our place in the world in the broader context of community and society, which, he claimed, "fosters a normative egocentricity that may contribute to self-constriction and alienation from self and other." The alternative proposed by Rubin is a "non-self-centered subjectivity," that is, "a non-self-preoccupied state of being" (p. 126), which is manifested in openness to the other and to the surrounding community. According to Rubin, the use of the word "object" in psychoanalytic theory to denote the other reflects its reductive view of the other and the relationships with the other:

> Psychoanalysis's impoverished view of relationships may be related to its narcissistic view of the self. It may not be accidental that psychoanalysis calls the other an "object" and relations with others "object relations." The word *object* connotes a thing and predisposes one to adopt a depersonalized view . . . and narcissistic relation to others.
>
> (pp. 133–134)

The narcissistic bias underlying psychoanalysis is discussed hereinafter with reference to the leading theorists of mainstream psychoanalysis who shaped psychoanalytic thought over the years, specifically Freud, Winnicott, and Kohut, whose life stories as related to their personality characteristics, views, and theories are discussed in depth in Chapter 4.

According to Freud, humans are primarily driven by aggressive and sexual impulses. Yet while they are basically egocentric and antisocial, they have no choice but to compromise and adapt to their environment. "Thus social feeling is based upon the reversal of what was first a hostile feeling into a positively-toned tie of the nature of an identification" (Freud, 1921, p. 121). That is, Freud interpreted manifestations of empathy for others or sharing with others as a reaction formation against the opposite negative feelings of indifference and inconsideration. In this context, Strenger's (1989) view of Freudian hermeneutics of suspicion is noteworthy:

> Freud rarely accepts what the patient says at face value. . . . Excessive altruism is often nothing but a reaction formation against sadistic wishes,

> shrill moralism a defense against threatening sexual desire. Too much of what looks sublime is really covert fulfillment of infantile wishes.
>
> (p. 598)

In the Oedipal drama, which is at the core of Freud's drive theory, the mother and father are regarded as vague figures, perceived by the child as mere imaginary objects for the satisfaction of instinctual drives. There is no specific reference in Freudian theory to the unique personality of the parents nor to their real-life relationships with their children. The focus is on the child's inner world, on his phantasies, fears, and wishes rather than on his real-world interaction with his parents.

Likewise, Winnicott and Kohut underplayed the need for interpersonal relationships. While they both viewed the other as significant and essential, it was only insofar as the other supported the self and facilitated self-growth and self-development. Thus, Winnicott put the self, that is, the infant, at the center of his theory of the parent-infant relationship, while the other – "the good enough mother" – was assigned the task of caring for the infant, attending to his physical needs, providing mirroring, sharing his infantile illusion of omnipotence, offering a nonintrusive presence, and so on. The significance of interpersonal relationships per se, irrespective of the fulfillment of needs, is hardly, if at all, referred to in Winnicott's writings. The only exception is an observation incidentally made by Winnicott and cited by Reeves (2004, p. 427) in his article on the Winnicott enigma:

> So many of my friends and contemporaries died in the first World War, and I have never been free from the feeling that my being alive is a facet of some one thing of which their deaths can be seen as other facets: some huge crystal, a body with integrity and shape intrinsical in it.
>
> (qtd. in C. Winnicott 1990, 6)

Commenting on Winnicott's atypical observation, Reeves (2004) noted:

> Again, this is unusual in that it appears to be the only occasion on which Winnicott describes the experience of "being alive" in terms of a sense of belonging to some larger unity – "a crystal." Elsewhere, it was his habit to attend to the very opposite characteristics of aliveness, namely, unity, integrity, and the sense of "being in one's own body," all of these phrases emphasizing the individual rather than the communal aspect of one's sense of one's own existence.
>
> (p. 428)

That is, the exception proves the rule. The observation by Winnicott is indeed exceptional given his view of human nature as driven by the fundamental need for personal self-realization and creative self-expression and his derogatory statements on communality as opposed to individuality (Winnicott, 1971):

> One could suppose that before a certain era, say a thousand years ago, only a very few people lived creatively. . . . To explain this one would have to say that before a certain date it is possible that there was only very exceptionally a man or woman who achieved unit status in personal development. Before a certain date the vast millions of the world of human beings quite possibly never found or certainly soon lost at the end of infancy or childhood their sense of being individuals. . . . We cannot easily identify ourselves with men and women of early times who so identified themselves with the community and with nature.
>
> (p. 70)

Orange (2011) criticized the individualistic position of Winnicott and his focus on individual self-realization and expression of the authentic self as the essence of life. Like Orange, I believe that the quest for self-realization and expression of the authentic self is not necessarily innate or universal, but rather reflects the norms and values of Western culture. As noted by Orange, and likewise by Rubin (1998), there are cultures that value communality and familial and communal conformity above individual self-realization. In contrast, Bollas (1989/2018), like other Winnicottians, highlighted the realization of the true self, or the *human idiom*, as he called it, as essential to personal growth as well as to the psychoanalytic process. And like Winnicott, Bollas believed that aloneness rather than interpersonal engagement was fundamental to human existence. "In our true self we are essentially alone . . . the absolute core of one's being is a wordless, imageless solitude. . . . In some respects, psychoanalysis is a place for the experiencing of essential aloneness" (p. 17).

Similarly, the self and self-realization are at the core of Kohut's theory of self-psychology. With reference to the essential role of self-realization in the human psyche, Kohut (1985) noted:

> The entire life cycle is implied as the self's nuclear program is laid down in an individual. The nonfulfillment of that program is evoked in anticipation by the hopeless and depressed child, who then turns to pleasure gain rather than to the fulfillment of the program.
>
> (p. 216)

The self was conceived by Kohut (1977) as "the center of the individual's psychological universe" (p. 311), while the other was primarily seen as an object designed to serve the self and actually, as part of the self rather than as separate from the self – a view aptly captured in the concept of *selfobject* coined by Kohut. Thus, the other, or *selfobject*, is supposed to enable the development and preservation of the self, mainly by fulfilling the narcissistic needs of the self, that is, mirroring, idealization, and twinship. At the same time, in contrast to Freud, who regarded adaptation to social and cultural norms and values as an undesirable yet inevitable compromise, Kohut believed that the cultural and social environment was of significance to individual development and experience. However, Kohut referred to the sociocultural milieu in terms of its contribution to enriching the self and promoting self-expression and self-cohesion (e.g., through involvement in cultural creativity or adherence to social and cultural values, inter alia, by admiration of role models) rather than in the context of social engagement, extroversion, openness to the other, interpersonal involvement, or close emotional relationships. Ornstein (1991), who was one of Kohut's followers and his partner in the development of self psychology, found it necessary to clarify why self psychology was not an object relations theory but rather a theory focused on the self and "on subjective experience (or self-experience), which includes the experiencing of the other as a selfobject" (p. 28). A change of approach, slight as it might have been, can be discerned in Kohut's (1984) last, posthumously published book. As noted by Togashi and Kottler (2021), while in his earlier writings Kohut (1968, 1971/2009) conceptualized the twinship experience as an experience of essential alikeness to the other that served the need for building and sustaining a cohesive self, toward the end of his life, he shifted focus and reconceptualized twinship as an essentially relational experience of being human among other human beings. However, Kohut (1984) did not expand on the point further than to say:

> The mere presence of people in a child's surroundings – their voices and body odors, the emotions they express, the noises they produce as they engage in human activities, the specific aroma of the foods they prepare and eat – creates a security in the child, a sense of belonging and participating, that cannot be explained in terms of a mirroring response or a merger with ideals. Instead, these feelings derive from confirmation of the feeling that one is a human being among other human beings.
>
> (pp. 199–200)

The narcissistic bias underlying the theories of Freud, Winnicott, and Kohut, as reflected in their focus on the self and the needs of the self and their failure to acknowledge the fundamental significance of communality, social ties, and close interpersonal relationships per se, is similarly manifest in the writings and concepts of other prominent theorists of mainstream psychoanalysis, first and foremost those associated with the school of ego psychology led by Anna Freud, who carried on her father's legacy, and including, among others, Heinz Hartmann, Edith Jacobson, and Margaret Mahler. Commenting on the focus of ego psychology on the self and self-autonomy, Aron and Starr (2013) noted:

> Within the ego psychological framework, the achievement of autonomy was established as the highest goal for the individual. It was held that the ego could achieve autonomy not only from the drives but also from the environment. This double autonomy provided the ego with the capacity for adjustment and adaptation.
>
> (p. 121)

The overarching goal of the individual as perceived by ego psychology theorists, namely, development of self-concept and self-autonomy separately from the other, with the emphasis on separation rather than on the enjoyment derived from interpersonal involvement, attachment to the other, or intimacy with the other, is epitomized in the separation-individuation theory of child development (Mahler et al., 1975). According to Mahler, the newborn emerges into the world oblivious of his surroundings and goes through a series of phases, from the initial autistic phase, when the neonate is unresponsive to the outside human world, through the symbiotic phase of fusion with the mother or surrogate figure, when the infant is unaware of the mother as a unique individual, to the ultimate developmental phase and goal of mental separation from the mother figure and consolidation of individuality, that is, individuation. Thus, in fact, the emotional relationship with the mother is not considered significant in itself but only as far as it empowers and fuels the journey toward self-autonomy and consolidation of self-identity. Bowlby (1988), who is known for his theory of attachment and belief in the child's innate need for attachment to one main attachment figure, critically noted in this context:

> Mahler's theories of normal development, including her postulated normal phases of autism and symbiosis, are shown to rest not on observation but on preconceptions based on traditional psychoanalytic theory and, in doing so, to ignore almost entirely the remarkable body of new information about early infancy.
>
> (pp. 35–36)

Likewise, Benjamin (1990) was critical of Mahler's theory, which "took the perspective of the child's movement away from the mother toward separation and individuation rather than highlighting the equally important movement toward mutual recognition and attachment" (p. 182):

> Because separation-individuation theory is formulated in terms of ego and object, it does not fully realize its own contribution. In the ego-object perspective the child is the individual, seen as moving in a progression toward autonomy and separateness. The telos of this process is the creation of psychic structure through internalization of the object in the service of greater independence. . . . This perspective also misses the *pleasure* of the evolving relationship with a partner from whom one knows how to elicit a response, but whose responses are not entirely predictable and assimilable to internal fantasy. The idea of pleasure was lost when ego psychology put the id on the backburner, but it might be restored by recognizing the subjectivity of the other.
>
> (pp. 186–187)

Other proponents of mainstream psychoanalysis transcended the narrow perspective of individualism and considered the individual in the broader context of the sociocultural environment. Thus, for instance, Erikson (1950/1963) highlighted the relation of the individual to society and thereby opened the door to a new perspective on the central role of interpersonal relationships in the human psyche. However, his theory is primarily concerned with the psychosocial development of the ego, namely, the self, and the developmental stages it undergoes through life rather than with the fundamental significance of interpersonal relationships as such. In the spirit of the ego psychology school with which he was associated, Erikson emphasized the role of the progress toward self-autonomy, the striving for initiative, and the consolidation of identity in the development of the ego. While he did discuss the ability to establish a close intimate relationship with the other, it was exclusively with reference to the young adulthood stage of development rather than from the broad perspective of human psychology. It is worth mentioning in this context that Mitchell and Black (1995/2016) chose to discuss Erikson's psychosocial development theory along with Kohut's theory of self-psychology under the heading "Psychologies of Identity and Self: Erik Erikson and Heinz Kohut" (p. 139). Erikson's focus on the self, self-definition, self-autonomy, self-development, and self-realization was criticized by Rubin (1998) as reflecting a Western-centric cultural bias:

> Erikson's account both superimposes concerns that may be more salient to males in the United States onto men and women from India and Japan and neglects what seems central to Indian and Japanese children. . . . But conceptions of the self are not . . . universal, transcultural, or transhistorical. Different societies construe selfhood in different ways.
>
> (p. 72)

Indeed, as noted by Rubin, ethnographic studies show that non-Western cultures place greater value on interpersonal relationships and mutual commitment than on self-autonomy or self-realization.

Similarly, the theorists associated with the object relations school, notably Melanie Klein and Otto Kernberg, focused in their writings on the relationships between self and object, seen as primarily aimed at the satisfaction of instinctual drives, as well as on the related intrapsychic dynamics (the conflicts, anxieties, and feelings of guilt induced by such instinctual desires) while failing to place due emphasis on the fundamental significance of emotional attachment, love feelings, and interpersonal relationships per se, irrespective of impulse gratification or need fulfillment. Elaborating on the early stages of infantile development, Klein (1957/2011) described the infant's tumultuous phantasy life as "being rooted in the instincts" (p. 58) and driven by the need for instinctual satisfaction rather than by the quest for emotional attachment. She painted a dark picture of the infant's ambivalent love-hate relationship with the mother, who is alternately perceived as a good (gratifying) or a bad (frustrating) object (the mother's breast), while the bad mother, imagined as a menacing monstrous figure, is looming over, giving rise to anxiety, death wish, envy, jealousy, and greed. However, the idea that the infant's unconscious intrapsychic dynamics is dominated by such morbid paranoid phantasies, which characterize psychotic illnesses in adult life, seems implausible, certainly when talking about a mentally healthy infant growing up in a loving and secure parental environment.

Bion, who underwent training analysis with Klein and built and expanded on her concepts, likewise focused on the inner world of the individual and his primitive unconscious phantasies while underestimating the fundamental significance of close interpersonal relationships. His shortsighted view of the significance of emotional attachment to an attachment figure is illustrated in his unsettling reaction to Robertson's film *A Two-Year-Old Goes to Hospital*. As related by Eagle (2013, citing Holmes, 1995), Bion ascribed the distress of the little girl to her envy of her mother's pregnancy, disregarding her sadness, loneliness, and fears as she was left on her own in hospital, away from her mother.

Drawing to a large extent on Freud's drive theory and Klein's object relations theory, Kernberg (1975), too, focused on the personality structure, the self-structure, and specifically the internalized representations of self and object and the relationships between self and object (whether colored by a positive, ideal affect or by a negative, distressing affect), which he regarded as the basic building blocks of the psyche. According to Kernberg, the drama taking place in the inner theater of the mind revolves around aggressive and sexual impulses (originating in the affects), which are manifested in interpersonal relationships throughout life as an inseparable part of the internalized representations of self and object and the relationships between self and object.[1] Furthermore, while Kernberg acknowledged the role of close interpersonal relationships and emotional attachment in the human psyche, he considered it of secondary importance to the instinctual vicissitudes. His model of the psyche is reflected in his psychotherapeutic strategy. As noted by Mitchell and Black (1995/2016), Kernberg "has maintained a steadfast commitment to the classical clinical principle of the centrality of interpretations in generating meaningful change" (p. 172), whereby the therapist is put in the neutral, uninvolved, interpretive position while the patient's projections of unacceptable desires, thoughts, and feelings, rather than his real-life relationships, whether with the therapist or outside the therapeutic setting, take center stage. What is more, his interpretations were based to a large extent on classical concepts related to the Oedipal complex – the aggressive and sexual impulses, envy, desire, and guilt – while overlooking the innate human need for social relatedness and the implications of the presence or absence of close interpersonal relationships in the life of the patient.

This brief review highlights the predominant focus of psychoanalytic theory on the self and its needs and its failure to place due emphasis on interpersonal relationships, which are generally perceived as significant only to the extent that they serve the self and meet its needs, fulfilling the functions of holding, containing, and mirroring, providing an object for projection and impulse gratification or object-images for internalization and thereby consolidation of the self. At the same time, the fundamental innate need for interpersonal involvement and affective bonding irrespective of impulse gratification or need fulfillment has not been duly considered. Moreover, the relationships addressed in psychoanalytic theory are unilateral for the most part, with the focus on the needs of the infant or child and their fulfillment by parental objects, while the unique personality and subjective world of the parent are generally absent from the equation. Last but not least, psychoanalytic theory has hardly, if at all, dealt with close relationships between siblings (beyond sheer envy, for instance) or with intimate couple relationships. On the whole, the significance of close intimate relationships per se, irrespective of any need they may fulfill, and the fundamental centrality of interpersonal relationships in the human psyche have been disregarded in psychoanalytic thought.

Inevitably, the focus on the self has had far-reaching implications for clinical practice, first and foremost as regards the goals set for the psychoanalytic process. For years, psychoanalysis was primarily concerned with the evocation of deep-seated wishes, desires, and needs, bringing to the surface repressed mental content, enhancing expression of the authentic self, offering an opportunity for corrective emotional experience through reenactment of early childhood traumas, transmuting internalized self- and object-images, improving self-esteem, enriching and diversifying the self, developing self-autonomy and self-differentiation, and so on. Focused on the self, these were all perceived as the overarching goals of psychoanalysis. At the same time, the nature of the patient's interpersonal relationships and related intrapsychic dynamics (e.g., avoidance of social and communal engagement, intimacy anxiety and the need to keep emotional distance, abandonment anxiety, or unprocessed grief) were not given due emphasis in the psychoanalytic setting. The advocates of traditional psychoanalytic practice would argue that constructive involvement in interpersonal relationships, whether close and intimate or social and communal, could be achieved as a by-product of self-development. However, I believe that while various aspects of the personality may be impressively developed, the capacity for good and satisfying interpersonal relationships could still be significantly inhibited, and given the fundamental centrality of interpersonal relationships in the human psyche, this would call for dedicated, specifically focused psychotherapeutic intervention. Yet the psychoanalytic discourse and clinical practice centered on the phantasy life of the individual rather than on his real-life events and relationships with real-life figures, whether past or present. Thus, formative life events in adulthood or even traumatic experiences, such as war, rape, social persecution, or brutal expatriation, were considered to be of less relevance. The primary focus of psychoanalytic practice on the patient's mental world rather than on his real-life relationships in or out of the therapeutic setting is reflected in the traditional psychoanalytic technique where the patient reclines on a sofa while the therapist sits out of sight, with no eye contact between the two, interpreting the patient's projections. This procedure, a vestige of the Freudian psychoanalytic approach that is still used by present-day psychoanalysts, even those who are aware of the importance of mutuality in psychoanalysis, is liable to encourage narcissistic-schizoid withdrawal into an inner world and thereby reinforce the preoccupation with the self (see Chapter 3 for an in-depth discussion of schizoidism as a core feature of the narcissistic personality). Freud himself admitted that he had difficulty being looked at by his patients for hours a day – that is, difficulty dealing with close human relationships. Aron (1996), who is known for his contribution to relational psychoanalysis, noted in this context, "There have been times when patients have told me how isolated they have felt on the couch" (p. 142). Psychoanalysis, taking place several times a week over long years, offers the patient an alternate reality focused on the self rather than on real-life relationships, whether between therapist and patient or between the patient and his surroundings – a form of escapism from the real world, where he would ultimately have to cope on his own.

The preoccupation with the self and reductive view of the other, the significance of the other, and the need for the other manifest in psychoanalytic theory and practice are characteristic of the narcissistic personality. Serving as a narcissistic self-protective shield, the reductive view of the other is closely associated with narcissistic grandiosity, that is, with a sense of superiority and omnipotence (as discussed at length in Chapter 3). Of special interest in this context is the reference by Aron and Starr (2013) as well as by Rubin (1998) to the air of superiority and the patronizing and even hostile attitude displayed for years by leading psychoanalysts and the psychoanalytic community in general toward women, minority groups, dissident thinkers, and divergent psychoanalytic practices, which further demonstrate the entrenched narcissistic position of the psychoanalytic establishment. Aron and Starr (2013) enlarged on the topic with reference to the post–World War II psychoanalytic scene, the heyday of ego psychology in the United States, "a time of great confidence in the profession," when "psychoanalysis exuded a sense of certainty and control" (p. 124). As noted by the authors, the psychoanalytic community of that era was dominated by a male majority whose members saw themselves as omnipotent figures, the representatives of the civilized, successful, advanced sectors of society, by far superior to the lesser sectors of women and various minorities. Furthermore, "psychoanalysis was thought to be pure gold, of greater value" (p. 202) than psychotherapy and other clinical practices. This supercilious attitude was clearly evident in the therapeutic setting as well, where the patient was viewed as childish and pathological while the analyst was in the authoritative, omniscient position. The omnipotent status of the psychoanalytic establishment was variously reflected in American culture, for instance, in the comic book series published at the time, which portrayed the analyst as an all-powerful superhero, "the Superman of the Mind . . . a powerful redeemer" (pp. 166–167), capable of resolving any case in no time. Yet as Aron and Starr observed, the arrogant attitude of the psychoanalytic establishment adversely affected the public at large and, in particular, women, homosexuals, and ethnic minorities:

> How many women were encouraged to stay home rather than work because of the use and misuse of analytic theories of gender and sexuality? How much harm was caused to people's marriages and families because analysts, endorsed by the authority of Freud and science, used analytic theory to encourage conservative and stereotyped gender norms?. . . Psychoanalysis' premise of a psychological cause for almost every ailment caused serious harm to families. Many parents were led to believe or were told outright that their children's difficulties, such as autism, learning disabilities, and behavioral problems, were caused by parental psychopathology. . . . Psychoanalysis blamed parents for children's schizophrenia (recall the famous "schizophrenogenic mother") and autism ("icebox parents").
>
> (pp. 13–14)

That said, it should be noted that psychoanalytic theory has offered invaluable insights into our understanding of human psychology, highlighting the significance of the unconscious and its deep-seated conflicts, anxieties, phantasies, dreams, wishes, desires, and complex mental processes. It has thereby contributed to legitimating individualism in Western culture, advocating the right to personal well-being, self-development, and self-realization. However, the narcissistic position displayed by psychoanalysis through the years and to a certain extent to this very day has shifted the balance to a disproportionate emphasis on the aspect of self-definition (as coined by Blatt) and excessive preoccupation with the self, in both theory and practice, while the fundamental centrality of interpersonal relationships in the human psyche has been played down and largely disregarded.

The big question

One may wonder why most theorists associated with mainstream psychoanalysis have chosen to present the other as an indistinct figure with no real significance in itself and disregard the innate human need for relatedness to the other. Why have they been blind to the fundamental role of interpersonal relationships in the human psyche, apart from and irrespective of the fulfillment of needs? Why have they failed to recognize the essential meaning of affective relationships and emotional attachment to a unique significant other as a primary phenomenon and address the related complex intrapsychic dynamics?[2] Aron and Starr (2013) pointed to the historical and cultural factors that influenced and shaped the narcissistic position of the pioneers of psychoanalysis, this, with reference to the grandiose aspect of narcissism and its self-protective role in maintaining a superior and invulnerable self-image. Thus, for instance, as noted by the authors, the post–World War II generation of psychoanalysts, who were, for the most part, Jewish émigrés traumatized by the horrors of war, used manic defense mechanisms against the trauma and loss in repudiation of their vulnerability. In this context, Aron and Starr observed (citing Klein, 1935 and Hinshelwood, 1989), "Manic defense is characterized by denial, omnipotence, disparagement or devaluation, contempt, triumph over the object, and omnipotent control. . . . All of these elements were characteristic of American psychoanalysis after the war" (p. 123).

While Aron and Starr (2013) highlighted general historical and cultural factors as contributing to the underlying narcissistic bias of psychoanalysis, this book turns the spotlight on the personal factors that shaped the narcissistic personality of the founding fathers of psychoanalysis – Freud, Winnicott, and Kohut. It is argued that their narcissistic personality traits colored their thinking in various ways, in particular, as reflected in the focus on the self (or as alternatively referred to, the ego) in their theories and in their failure to take due account of the fundamental significance of interpersonal relationships and their key role in the organization of the human psyche. The impact of personal and subjective factors on the formulation of theory is illustrated in the next chapter. In that context, it is observed that the impact of the narcissistic personality on theory, specifically psychoanalytic theory, goes even deeper and could thus undermine its validity and universal applicability.

Notes

1 Rather than independently of the internalized representations of self and object and the relationships between self and object, as suggested by Freud.
2 It should be noted though that as previously observed and discussed in detail in Chapter 6, the intersubjective relational approach highlights the importance of interpersonal relationships as central to the human psyche.

References

Aron, L. (1996). *A meeting of minds: Mutuality in psychoanalysis*. The Analytic Press. https://read.amazon.com/?asin=B0B9KHXHZ1&ref_=kwl_kr_iv_rec_3
Aron, L., & Starr, K. (2013). *A psychotherapy for the people: Toward a progressive psychoanalysis*. Routledge/Taylor & Francis Group.
Bakan, D. (1966). *The duality of human existence: Isolation and communion in Western man*. Beacon Press.
Benjamin, J. (1990). Recognition and destruction: An outline of intersubjectivity. In S. A. Mitchell & L. Aron (Eds.), *Relational psychoanalysis: The emergence of a tradition* (pp. 181–210). Routledge.
Blatt, S. J. (2008). *Polarities of experience: Relatedness and self-definition in personality development, psychopathology, and the therapeutic process*. American Psychological Association.
Bollas, C. (2018). *Forces of destiny: Psychoanalysis and human idiom*. Routledge. https://doi.org/10.4324/9781315533414 (Original work published 1989)
Bowlby, J. (1988). *A secure base: Parent-child attachment and healthy human development*. Basic Books.
Bowles, S. (2006). Group competition, reproductive leveling, and the evolution of human altruism. *Science, 314*(5805), 1569–1572.
Eagle, M. N. (2013). *Attachment and psychoanalysis: Theory, research, and clinical implications*. Guilford Press.
Erikson, E. H. (1963). *Childhood and society* (2nd ed.). Norton. (Original work published 1950)

Freud, S. (1921). *Group psychology and the analysis of the ego* (J. Strachey, Ed. & Trans., Standard Edition, Vol. 18, pp. 65–144). The International Psychoanalytical Library.
Kernberg, O. F. (1975). *Borderline conditions and pathological narcissism*. Rowman & Littlefield. https://read.amazon.com/?asin=B00BZAMWA0&ref_=kwl_kr_iv_rec_23
Klein, M. (2011). *Envy and gratitude and other works 1946–1963*. Random House. (Original work published 1957)
Kohut, H. (1977). *The restoration of the self*. International Universities Press.
Kohut, H. (1984). *How does analysis cure?* (A. Goldberg, Ed., with P. E. Stepansky). The University of Chicago Press. https://read.amazon.com/?asin=B015KJZF8M&ref_=kwl_kr_iv_rec_1
Kohut, H. (1985). *Self psychology and the humanities: Reflections on a new psychoanalytic approach* (C. B. Strozier, Ed.). Norton.
Mahler, M. S., Pine, F., & Bergman, A. (1975). *The psychological birth of the human infant: Symbiosis and individuation*. Routledge. https://doi.org/10.4324/9780429482915
Mitchell, S. A. (2023). *Relationality: From attachment to intersubjectivity*. Routledge. https://read.amazon.com/?asin=B0B92S5PVW&ref_=kwl_kr_iv_rec_3 (Original work published 2000)
Mitchell, S. A., & Black, M. J. (2016). *Freud and beyond: A history of modern psychoanalytic thought*. Basic Books. https://read.amazon.com/?asin=B06XBVPQGS&ref_=kwl_kr_iv_rec_1 (Original work published 1995)
Orange, D. M. (2011). *The suffering stranger: Hermeneutics for everyday clinical practice*. Routledge.
Ornstein, P. H. (1991). Why self psychology is not an object relations theory: Clinical and theoretical considerations. In A. Goldberg (Ed.), *The evolution of self psychology: Progress in self psychology* (Vol. 7, pp. 17–29). The Analytic Press.
Reeves, C. (2004). On being "intrinsical": A Winnicott enigma. *American Imago, 61*(4), 427–455.
Rubin, J. B. (1998). *A psychoanalysis for our time: Exploring the blindness of the seeing I*. New York University Press.
Strenger, C. (1989). The classic and the romantic vision in psychoanalysis. *The International Journal of Psychoanalysis, 70*(4), 593–610.
Togashi, K., & Kottler, A. (2021). From a cohesive self to a relational being: The evolution of the psychology of the self to the psychology of being human. *Psychoanalytic Inquiry, 41*(3), 187–198. https://doi.org/10.1080/07351690.2021.1886825
Winnicott, D. W. (1971). *Playing and reality*. Tavistock Publications.

2 The inevitable impact of personal and subjective factors on personality theories

> "In psychology, the means by which you study the psyche is the psyche itself . . . the observer is the observed. The psyche is not only the object, but also the subject of our science."
>
> (Jung, 1968, as cited by Atwood & Stolorow, 1993, p. 6)

Personality theories are inevitably colored by the personal life history and subjective world of the theorist (Atwood & Stolorow, 1993; Renik, 2006; Symington & Symington, 1996). Formative life experiences as well as cultural and social influences are destined to leave an indelible mark on the personality, views, and beliefs of the theorist and ultimately shape his theory. Seeking to understand human nature, the theorist tends to draw on his personal life experience and focus on specific psychological phenomena and intrapsychic processes that concern him personally, evoking his own deep-seated needs, desires, anxieties, and enduring vulnerabilities. Thus, for instance, the theorist may conceive of the mind as an apparatus driven by an instinctually based psychic energy and trace the origin of anxiety to guilt over taboo impulses, as suggested by Freud. Others may be preoccupied with existential issues of self-realization and expression of the authentic self and see the potential disintegration of the self as the source of human anxiety, as perceived by Winnicott and Kohut. Furthermore, mental health criteria, unlike physical health measures, are not unequivocally defined. Thus, we may wonder whether the ability to love and to work indeed distinguishes a psychologically healthy person and if the willingness to give up infantile wishes and fantasies and settle for a humdrum life is a measure of mental health, as maintained by Freud, or whether it is rather the ability to feel alive, give free rein to the imagination, unlock creativity, and strive for expression of the authentic self, as suggested by Winnicott. Clinical practices may be likewise influenced by the theorist's subjective perspectives and needs. One may wonder whether the evocation of unconscious mental content and repressed memories and the insights thereby gained are of prime importance in the psychoanalytic process or if it is rather the patient-therapist relationship that makes a difference and the empathy, containment, and corrective

DOI: 10.4324/9781003538295-2

emotional experience offered by the therapist that are of real significance. The diverse answers offered by various personality theorists to these and other questions are influenced by the unique personality and subjective world of the theorist, as shaped by his personal life experience. Based on psychobiographical analyses of Sigmund Freud, Carl Jung, Wilhelm Reich, and Otto Rank, Atwood and Stolorow (1993) sought to trace the subjective origins of the theories of these pioneers of psychoanalysis. As noted by the authors, there are organizing principles, that is, perceptual templates, developed in early childhood through which the individual perceives the self and the other and the relationships between self and other and interprets internal and external reality later on in life. Thus, the portrayal of the mother in the Freudian Oedipal drama as the object of her son's desire and love, in contrast to the father, who is depicted as a threatening rival, triggering castration anxiety and provoking ambivalent feelings, is attributed by the authors to Freud's abandonment anxiety. As related, Freud went through a series of abandonment experiences, the first, when he was just over a year and a half old, upon the death of his baby brother, Julius. With his mother overcome by grief, Freud most probably felt emotionally abandoned, a feeling that only intensified when his five sisters and little brother, Alexander, were born one after the other, taking up his mother's time and attention. At the age of two and a half years, Freud experienced another traumatic abandonment upon the sudden disappearance of a significant attachment figure, his nanny, who was indicted on theft charges and sentenced to prison time. According to the authors, Freud was overwhelmed by anxiety, and fearing that he would be abandoned once again, he resorted to denial of his negative feelings toward his mother lest they jeopardize his precarious relationship with her. Citing Freud as observing that the relationship between mother and son is the most perfect of all human relationships, the authors noted that it pointed to his defensive idealization of the maternal figure, universalized by him with reference to mother-son relationships in general.

Another illustrative case discussed by Atwood and Stolorow (1993) concerns the key concepts introduced by Jung – individuation and the collective unconscious – and their subjective origins in his formative childhood experiences and personality. According to Jung (1961/1989), individuation is a developmental process characterized by acknowledgment and integration of the different and, at times, conflicting parts of the self, whereby the individual can attain a sense of wholeness and oneness of the self. This integrative process is at the core of Jungian analytical psychotherapy, which Jung himself was in need of, as he openly acknowledged, being aware of his dissociated personality:

> Somewhere deep in the background I always knew that I was two persons. One was the son of my parents, who went to school and was less intelligent, attentive, hard-working, decent, and clean than many other boys. The other was grown up – old, in fact – skeptical, mistrustful,

> remote from the world of men, but close to nature, the earth, the sun, the moon, the weather, all living creatures, and above all close to the night, to dreams, and to whatever "God" worked directly in him.
>
> (pp. 62–63)

As for the collective unconscious, conceived by Jung as a part of the unconscious comprising a set of inherited archetypes shared by all humans and representing aspects of the psyche derived from the accumulated experience of the human race (including the mother figure, the trickster, and the shadow, which represents the darker, unacceptable aspect of the human psyche), Atwood and Stolorow (1993) traced this concept of universality and shared human experience to Jung's childhood feelings of loneliness, eccentricity, and exclusion and his need for belonging, sharing and connecting with other human beings.

It is no wonder that Freud, in particular, was featured in various psychobiographical analyses. Aron and Starr (2013) discussed the life story of Freud and its impact on his personality and theory against the broad cultural and historical background of the time, specifically with reference to the anti-Semitism of that era. According to the authors, the Freudian Oedipal drama can be understood in light of the then prevalent binary ideology, manifested, inter alia, in anti-Semitism and misogyny, which divided the world into those who were worth more and those who were worth less. Gentile white males were considered superior, while Jewish men were deemed not only inferior but also effeminate, passive, immoral, and irrational (like women). Freud sought to shake off the image of the Jew as castrated (having undergone circumcision) and perversely incestuous (perceived as such given the adherence of the Jews throughout history to their distinct identity and in-community marriage tradition, adopted in the face of the danger of assimilation). The Oedipus complex as presented in the Freudian Oedipal drama, whereby the son's incestuous desire for the mother and related castration anxiety are universal and hence not necessarily unique to Jews, can thus be seen as reflecting a defensive position taken by Freud. At the same time, his theory of penis envy enabled him to project onto women his feelings of inferiority and vulnerability as a Jew, seen as a defective castrated male in the virulent anti-Semitic Viennese society of his time.

The life stories of Winnicott and Kohut as related to their personalities and theories were also variously discussed in the literature. Rodman (2003), the biographer of Winnicott, traced the concept of the authentic self, a key concept in Winnicottian theory, to Winnicott's difficulty in expressing his own authentic self, noting that he had to sacrifice his true self to please his depressive mother. A childhood episode related by Rodman is illustrative of Winnicott's lifelong search for authentic self-expression. As the story goes, at the age of nine, Winnicott looked at the mirror and decided that he was "too nice" (p. 19). Displeased with the image of an ingratiating child, Winnicott deliberately adopted an unruly and defiant stance and was subsequently sent by his concerned father to a prestigious boarding school to keep him away from bad company. Yet while apparently wild and rebellious, Winnicott could not really behave impolitely or treat others aggressively. Throughout life, he struggled for expression of his true self and thus saw the quest for expression of the authentic self as a universal human endeavor.

In an article dealing with Kohut's erasure of the analyst's trauma, Philipson (2017) discussed his derogatory view of "social psychology," as he termed it, and its superficial focus on external social and cultural factors, the way he saw it, tracing it to his Holocaust trauma. Kohut, a Jew by origin, had to escape Vienna, his beloved city, leaving behind a way of life and the cherished Viennese culture of operas, concerts, theater shows, and coffee houses that were so significant to him and defined his innermost identity. The move to the United States as an émigré fleeing the horrors of war and the need to build up his life again were unbearably traumatic for him, so much so that he could not acknowledge the devastating impact of the war on his own life or, for that matter, on the lives of his patients. Denying the trauma, Kohut chose to focus in his theory and clinical practice on early childhood experiences, psychological development, relationships with parental figures, and the extent to which they fulfilled or failed to fulfill the child's narcissistic needs rather than deal with traumatic social and historical events, whether traumatic childhood events or those that occurred later on in life, which in either case had a deep and lasting impact on the personality.

Freud, Winnicott, and Kohut themselves engaged in psychobiographical analysis of other prominent figures. Freud, the founding father of psychoanalysis, set out to explore other realms. Intrigued by "the great personages of humanity," Freud (1916/2010) chose to focus on the life and art of Leonardo da Vinci, "one of the greatest men of the Italian Renaissance" (Chapter I). In a psychoanalytic study of Leonardo da Vinci's life story and its impact on his great works of art, specifically the *Mona Lisa*, Freud cited an early childhood memory of Leonardo or, more precisely, a phantasy of the artist, as told by him:

> It seems that it had been destined before that I should occupy myself so thoroughly with the vulture, for it comes to my mind as a very early memory, when I was still in the cradle, a vulture came down to me, he opened my mouth with his tail and struck me a few times with his tail against my lips. (Chapter II)

Freud interpreted the vulture phantasy, alluding to its undertones of homosexuality, as symbolizing the deep love relationship between Leonardo and his mother – indeed, too intimate a relationship, considered by Freud the main cause of Leonardo's homosexuality (as noted by Freud, the mother figure was represented as a vulture in sacred Egyptian hieroglyphs). According to Freud, the enigmatic and seductive *Mona Lisa* was actually a portrait of Leonardo's mother, illustrating the impact of the artist's subjective world on his artistic creation. Yet the subjectivity of the personality theorist, unlike that of the artist, has far-reaching implications that are liable to be problematic, as noted in Chapter 1 and discussed at more length hereinafter.

Winnicott (1964) offered a psychobiographical analysis of Jung in his review of Jung's (1961/1989) partly autobiographical book *Memories, Dreams, Reflections*. As noted by Winnicott (1964), "Jung, in describing himself, gives us a picture of childhood schizophrenia" (p. 450). Tracing Jung's key theoretical concepts to his personality and personal life events, Winnicott attributed the focus on the collective unconscious in Jungian theory, highlighted at the expense of the personal unconscious, to Jung's split personality and defensive dissociation. By focusing on the collective unconscious, Jung was spared the need, as it were, for repression of painful and unacceptable mental content and its delegation to the personal unconscious. In contrast to the personal unconscious, the collective unconscious has no personally defensive role in Jungian theory, but rather serves as a universal frame of reference consisting of the inherited archetypes shared by all humans. Furthermore, the use of the mandala (a circular pattern of symbols) by Jung as a therapeutic means of promoting harmony and serenity was seen by Winnicott as reflecting "an obsessional flight from disintegration" (p. 454), and hence Jung's failure to cope with destructiveness and chaos.

Kohut discussed the personality and theory of Freud in several of his writings (1977, 1984, 1985), specifically with reference to Freud's belief that the evocation and acknowledgment of unconscious, repressed mental content is a key aspect of psychoanalytic therapy. According to Kohut, Freud had a real need to discover the truth, inspired by his childhood milieu as well as by contemporary cultural perceptions that championed the quest for the objective truth, and if something was withheld from him, he experienced it as an outrageous narcissistic injury.

These examples illustrate the need for analyzing and understanding the subjective world of the theorist and its impact on his theory so as to evaluate its validity and applicability. This is all the more true for theories that are likely to have far-reaching implications for the mental health and well-being of individuals seeking professional help. Theories concerning human nature, personality structure, and psychological needs propose not only abstract ideas that can be accepted or rejected but also guidelines for clinical practice that may be potentially harmful. Thus, as noted by Aron and Starr (2013), psychoanalytic practices adversely affected certain population groups, for instance, women and homosexuals, due to biased preconceptions. Given the inherent subjective bias of the theorist, the question then arises whether personality theories can be taken at face value and accepted as universally valid. Strozier (2001) addressed the question in his biography of Kohut. "Perhaps any thinker, especially a psychological one, draws on his or her own conflicts as the basis of insight. The question, however, is not whether theories are subjective but whether such insight can be generalized" (p. 260). In other words, Strozier assumes that the subjective experiential world of the theorist is a given and that its impact on theory is inevitable. The critical question then is to what extent the formative life events, the personality, and the subjectivity of the theorist are dominant and hence limit the generality of his theory. In this context, Strozier noted:

> Kohut, probably more than any other psychological theorist in recent decades, wrote in general about humans in ways that grew intimately out of his own experience . . . Sometimes, however, the self-referential quality of Kohut's writings limits the more general applicability of his psychology.
>
> (p. 260)

It may then be concluded that the subjectivity of psychological knowledge is inevitable and that the question we have to answer is whether the subjective bias underlying a personality theory is not too sweeping, to the exclusion of its generalization. Theorists associated with the intersubjective relational approach, who draw on postmodern epistemology, which argues that there can be no objective or absolute truth, may dismiss the question as irrelevant since no theory can be free of personal bias.[1] Moreover, they maintain that no personality theory laying claim to universal truth should be applied in clinical practice as each patient is a unique individual and hence cannot be understood unless considered individually through an ongoing dialogue. Thus, for instance, Orange (2011) was against the application of any theory whatsoever in the therapeutic setting or the use of any diagnostic criteria. Instead, Orange proposed "to contact and to understand the suffering other" (p. 4) directly, without any theoretical conceptualizations or classifications. The way patients are diagnosed, through the lens of theory, is seen by Orange as well as by other relational and intersubjective theorists as a reductionist practice that fits "the patient into our preformed or preconceived categories, diagnoses, and theories" (p. 188) and rules out an open and authentic human encounter between patient and clinician. I believe that a balanced therapeutic approach based on theoretical understanding of mental processes as well as on consideration of the patient's uniqueness and subjectivity would be more effective and beneficial. Thus, while drawing on the body of psychoanalytic knowledge and the theoretical, empirical, and clinical insights gained over the years in the psychological domain and in related disciplines, we should strive to develop a new approach that would promote our theoretical understanding of human psychology while encouraging a genuine and constructive human encounter with the individual patient. Bearing in mind the limitations posed by the theorist's subjectivity, the need for a more inclusive, in-depth, universally valid theory of human nature cannot be overestimated (Govrin, 2006). Indeed, the subjective experiential world of the theorist does not necessarily present an insurmountable obstacle. The tendency of personality theorists "to rely on their own lives as a primary source of empirical material" noted by Atwood and Stolorow

(1993, p. 6) could position them in a vantage point for the exploration of the psychological needs and mental processes shared by others. Obviously, the theorist should be aware of and acknowledge his own deep-seated anxieties and vulnerabilities. No less important are social engagement and involvement in close interpersonal relationships, through which the theorist can gain firsthand insights into human psychology. Interest in and openness to unfamiliar cultures and foreign people could further deepen the theorist's understanding of the human psyche. In the absence of these qualities, the universality of the proposed personality theory would inevitably be limited.

This book presents a critical review of psychoanalytic theory and its clinical implications viewed through the lens of narcissism. As argued (and discussed in more detail in Chapter 2), theorists with narcissistic personality traits are particularly prone to subjective bias. Tending to be self-centered, focused on their own needs and feelings and less so on others and, at times, unable to acknowledge and deal with their own vulnerabilities, they are often blind to major aspects of the human existence, specifically the fundamental centrality of interpersonal relationships and emotional attachment to a significant other in the psychodynamics of the individual. A similarly narcissistic position is manifested in their difficulty accepting the otherness of the other and adopting an open attitude toward people from other cultures or of other beliefs. Yet paradoxically, narcissistically biased theorists, more than others, are driven by their sense of grandiosity, high motivation, determination, courage, creativity, and inventiveness (Maccoby, 2004; Smith & Webster, 2018) and thus dare undertake ambitious projects, such as the formulation of a comprehensive and complex theory of the human psyche. Indeed, it is not by mere coincidence that Freud, Winnicott, and Kohut displayed prominent narcissistic personality traits. The core characteristics of the narcissistic personality are discussed in depth in the next chapter and their manifestation in the personality of each of these three leading figures in the development of psychoanalysis is illustrated, based on psychobiographical analysis, in Chapter 4.

Note

1 As discussed in more detail in Chapter 6.

References

Aron, L., & Starr, K. (2013). *A psychotherapy for the people: Toward a progressive psychoanalysis*. Routledge/Taylor & Francis Group.

Atwood, G. E., & Stolorow, R. D. (1993). *Faces in a cloud: Intersubjectivity in personality theory*. Jason Aronson.

Freud, S. (2010). *Leonardo da Vinci: A psychosexual study of an infantile reminiscence* (A. A. Brill, Trans.). www.bartleby.com/277/ (Original work published 1916)

Govrin, A. (2006). The dilemma of contemporary psychoanalysis: Toward a "knowing" post-postmodernism. *Journal of the American Psychoanalytic Association*, *54*(2), 507–535. https://doi.org/10.1177/00030651060540020801

Jung, C. G. (1989). *Memories, dreams, reflections.* (A. Jaffé, Ed.; R. Winston & C. Winston, Trans.; rev. ed.). Vintage Books. https://read.amazon.com/?asin=B004FYZK52&ref_=kwl_kr_iv_rec_2 (Original work published 1961)

Kohut, H. (1977). *The restoration of the self.* International Universities Press.

Kohut, H. (1984). *How does analysis cure?* (A. Goldberg, Ed., with P. E. Stepansky). The University of Chicago Press. https://read.amazon.com/?asin=B015KJZF8M&ref_=kwl_kr_iv_rec_1

Kohut, H. (1985). *Self psychology and the humanities: Reflections on a new psychoanalytic approach* (C. B. Strozier, Ed.). Norton.

Maccoby, M. (2004). Narcissistic leaders: The incredible pros, the inevitable cons. In *Leadership perspectives* (pp. 31–39). Routledge.

Orange, D. M. (2011). *The suffering stranger: Hermeneutics for everyday clinical practice*. Routledge.

Philipson, I. (2017). Fearing the theoretical other: The legacy of Kohut's erasure of the analyst's trauma. *Psychoanalysis, Self and Context, 12*(3), 211–220.

Renik, O. (2006). *Practical psychoanalysis for therapists and patients*. Other Press.

Rodman, F. R. (2003). *Winnicott: Life and work*. Perseus Publishing.

Smith, M. B., & Webster, B. D. (2018). Narcissus the innovator? The relationship between grandiose narcissism, innovation, and adaptability. *Personality and Individual Differences, 121*, 67–73.

Strozier, C. B. (2001). *Heinz Kohut: The making of a psychoanalyst*. Farrar, Straus, and Giroux.

Symington, J., & Symington, N. (1996). *The clinical thinking of Wilfred Bion*. Routledge.

Winnicott, D. W. (1964). Review of C. G. Jung, memories, dreams, reflections. *The International Journal of Psychoanalysis, 45*, 450–455.

3 The self-sufficient grandiose self

A discussion of narcissism

The narcissistic self-protective shield

Narcissism serves as a self-protective shield, reflected in grandiosity, schizoidism, and the difficulty acknowledging the otherness and separateness of the other, which are, as suggested, the three core features of the narcissistic personality.

Grandiosity

The well-known Greek myth of Narcissus tells the story of a beautiful youth whose dazzling beauty allured women, men, and nymphs alike. However, he was so self-absorbed that he remained unmoved by their advances and rejected them one after the other. Even the lovely nymph Echo could not tempt him. Repulsed by Narcissus, she pined away, heartbroken, with only the echo of her voice lingering behind. As for Narcissus, enchanted by his beauty, he fell in love with his own image, reflected in a pool of clear water that he chanced upon during his wanderings. But to his growing dismay, the object of his desire disappeared as he tried time and again to reach out and embrace it. His tragic end was predestined. According to one version of the myth, Narcissus drowned as he knelt to hug his reflection in the pool, and according to another version, unable to tear himself away from his image, he died of thirst, and as the story goes, he was transformed into the flower that bears his name.

The name of Narcissus lives on as a synonym for obsessive self-love and an inflated, superior, grandiose sense of self. Like Narcissus, narcissists are often endowed with exceptional qualities or abilities. Some are highly intelligent, while others have outstanding musical talent, excel in sports, or are otherwise gifted, displaying qualities and talents that enhance their superior, grandiose sense of self.

A patient of mine, a bright young woman with manifestly narcissistic personality traits, once told me in a condescending, matter of fact tone, "I am so bored with my friends. They don't challenge me intellectually. Only few people are as quick-thinking as I am or can understand complex concepts as

DOI: 10.4324/9781003538295-3

I do. My score in an IQ test that I took in third grade was above the top of the scale. There are maybe 5% of the population on par with me." And she was not far off. She is indeed exceptionally intelligent. However, her need to constantly compare herself with others and thereby maintain her inflated sense of self points to a defensive narcissistic personality pattern. Her self-identity is defensively reduced down to a single quality or ability, while other parts of her personality that may be perceived by her or by others as reflecting weakness or vulnerability are ignored and denied.

The *Diagnostic and Statistical Manual of Mental Disorders* (5th ed.; DSM-5; American Psychiatric Association, 2013), which uses phenomenological classification of personality traits and behaviors to diagnose mental disorders, highlights grandiosity as a key characteristic of the narcissistic personality. The diagnostic criteria for narcissistic personality disorder specified in the DSM-5 portray people with a grandiose sense of self-importance and arrogant behavior who are preoccupied with fantasies of unlimited success related to their unique qualities or abilities; who require excessive admiration, often using their personal charm to that end; and who believe that they are special and can only be understood by other special, gifted, or high-status people like them. While this description is partial and even superficial in that it leaves out other core characteristics of the narcissistic personality, which are discussed at length hereinafter, it emphasizes, and rightly so, the pervasive pattern of grandiosity, whether in fantasy or in behavior, typical of the narcissistic personality (Afek, 2018).

Already Freud (1914/1957) in his essay *On Narcissism: An Introduction* drew a direct line between narcissism and an inflated, illusory, and megalomaniac sense of self. It should be noted, though, that Freud saw narcissism as related to various phenomena, such as schizophrenia, dreams, homosexuality, and so on, rather than as associated with a specific personality structure. Yet his personality schema, whereby the ideal ego is depicted as the heir to infantile narcissism, that is, as that part of the personality that reflects the ideal image of a perfect self that one strives to emulate even though it can never be fully realized, indicates that Freud equated narcissism with a grandiose sense of self-perfection:

> This ideal ego is now the target of the self-love which was enjoyed in childhood by the actual ego. The subject's narcissism makes its appearance displaced on to this new ideal ego, which, like the infantile ego, finds itself possessed of every perfection that is of value. As always where the libido is concerned, man has here again shown himself incapable of giving up a satisfaction he had once enjoyed. He is not willing to forgo the narcissistic perfection of his childhood; and when, as he grows up, he is disturbed by the admonitions of others and by the awakening of his own critical judgement, so that he can no longer retain that perfection, he seeks to recover it in the new form of an ego ideal. What he projects before him as his ideal is the substitute for the lost narcissism of his childhood in which he was his own ideal.
>
> (p. 94)

Kernberg (1975) saw the grandiose self as a key defensive element at the core of narcissism. He attributed the pathological narcissistic personality structure to early childhood fears of potential abuse by a maternal figure perceived as menacing, whether due to feelings of aggression projected onto her or because of actual hostility, indifference, or neglect on her part. In either case, according to Kernberg, aspects of the actual self are fused with aspects of the ideal self and aspects of the ideal object to form an inflated, grandiose sense of self, which allows the narcissist a way out of dealing with his painful early childhood experiences. In the same vein, Masterson (1981/2013) and Rothstein (1984/1999) suggested, each in his own way, that narcissism was manifested in an illusive, omnipotent, ideal self-image attributable to defensive regression and traced back to frustrating relationships with the parental figure in the separation-individuation process.

Mitchell (1986) addressed the narcissistic illusion in his essay on the Greek myth of Daedalus and his son Icarus, who soared above Crete on wings made from feathers joined by wax to escape their captivity by King Minos, defying the laws of nature, an escapade that ended tragically when Icarus, who ignored his father's warnings and ventured higher and higher until his wings melted in the sun, fell to his death in the sea. Mitchell's discussion of this narcissistic display of grandiosity, hubris, and omnipotence demonstrates his view of grandiosity as directly linked to narcissism.

The illusory narcissistic experience of omnipotence is likewise exemplified by the fictional character of Peter Pan, the eternal boy who would not grow up, disregarding the limitations of age, the passing of time, and the finality of life. The Peter Pan syndrome, that is, the illusion of eternal youth, is typical of the narcissistic personality. It may be displayed in constant efforts to mask the telltale signs of age by plastic surgery or in denial of the reality of aging, for instance, by dodging the mirror and the withered image it reflects or by adopting an ostensibly youthful, free lifestyle, liberally indulging one's desires, avoiding having children, choosing much younger partners, and so on. The narcissistic refusal to acknowledge the passing of time is aptly captured in the celebrated novel by Oscar Wilde, which tells the story of Dorian Gray, who sells his soul for eternal youth and beauty. Dorian's wish to stay forever young and beautiful while his painted portrait, rather than he, will age and decay, is granted. As Dorian leads a debauched hedonistic life while retaining his youth and beauty, his portrait ages, turning into a hideous record of his depravity. Eventually, Dorian becomes aware of the deplorable immorality of his dissolute life, to which the painting bears witness, and rips his portrait in a moment of rage. He is found stabbed in the heart, a shriveled and withered old man, next to his image as a beautiful and charmingly attractive youth.

The narcissistic sense of grandiosity may also be reflected in an image of the self as an amorphous, godlike being with supernatural qualities. Bach (1985) described a case of a narcissistic patient who was alarmed to realize as a child, when returning home from the hospital with his parents and newly born baby sister, that he was not the omnipotent magical being he envisioned himself to be, but rather, just like his sister, a regular human being, born and going through the same developmental path as any other human being. One of my patients once told me that if he were to see himself walking down the street, he would wonder, "Who is this person?" He thus expressed his alienation and detachment from *that person*, who was walking along just like all other common human beings with common human qualities. Another patient of mine was enraged when I remarked in passing that she tended to take on the role of the funny clown in unfamiliar social settings. "I can be anything I fancy . . . I can be funny if I feel like it or just watch from the side . . . there's no need to classify me," she retorted angrily. Apparently unable to come to terms with her human limitations, she felt belittled and devalued when characterized, even if not necessarily negatively, in terms of specifically defined personality traits and resisted being typecast in a way perceived by her as detracting from her fantasized supernatural omnipotence. As noted by Bach, the narcissist finds it difficult to see himself as one integrated entity with clear-cut, well-defined boundaries and rather than facing his limitations, takes the subjective, fuzzy perspective of the self, which enables him to maintain his illusory grandiose sense of self-perfection.

Similarly typical of the grandiose narcissistic position is the sense of entitlement, the belief that one is special and therefore entitled to special privileges denied to others and exempt from conforming to norms and standards of behavior required of others. Freud (1916/1957) attributed such nonconforming behavior of persons with an "exceptional" personality feeling entitled to act immorally to strict discipline in childhood, perceived as unjustified.

While variously expressed, grandiosity is widely seen as a core characteristic of the narcissistic personality (Caligor, 2013; Diamond et al., 2013; Diamond et al., 2022; Horney, 1939/2000; Kernberg, 1975; Morf, 2006; Morf & Rhodewalt, 2001; Perry & Presniak, 2013; Symington, 1993). It is also considered the diagnostic hallmark of the narcissistic personality disorder, distinguishing it from other personality disorders (Diamond et al., 2022; Ronningstam & Gunderson, 1990; Sharp et al., 2015). Grandiosity may be readily identified when expressed by overtly displayed haughtiness and arrogance, by a condescending attitude toward others and disregard for others, or by the flaunting of an outstanding talent or quality, high status, exceptional achievements, and so on. It is less apparent when expressed in fantasies, delusions, or a covert sense of superiority and omnipotence. The diagnostic criteria of the DSM-5 have come under criticism for this very reason, as they rely on observable personality traits and behaviors and thus ignore a less known group of narcissists whose grandiosity is not openly manifested. Such narcissists have been variously referred to in the literature as vulnerable (Pincus et al., 2014), thin-skinned and hypersensitive (Rosenfeld, 1987), hypervigilant (Gabbard, 1989), or covert and shy (Ronningstam, 2005). They do not display an arrogant or condescending attitude, and in most cases, they are too embarrassed to show their sense of superiority and omnipotence. Rather, they appear to be modest, gentle, and reserved. They often fail to constructively cope with the challenges of interpersonal relationships and manage interpersonal conflicts and lack the confidence to carve out a place for themselves, be it at work or elsewhere, and they are thus less successful career-wise than the overtly grandiose narcissists. They may shut themselves up at home for hours or days on end, fantasizing about spectacular success as, for instance, writers, musicians, or software developers, and dreaming of attaining one day number one position in their area of accomplishment.

Other variants of narcissism discussed in the literature include malignant narcissism (Kernberg, 2007) and the related and, to a large extent, overlapping type of psychopathic narcissism (Ronningstam, 2005), both characterized by extreme aggression and, at times, even outright sadism, as displayed by murderous tyrants such as Adolf Hitler, Joseph Stalin, and Saddam Hussein. The destructive impact of malignant or psychopathic narcissism is otherwise shown in the case of pathologically narcissistic cult leaders, who unscrupulously use their charisma to subordinate, dominate, manipulate, and exploit their followers to satisfy their own needs and desires. A case in point is that of Keith Raniere, the leader of the purportedly self-improvement group NXIVM, who was convicted of physically, emotionally, sexually, and financially abusing his victims, as documented in the intriguing TV series *The Vow*. Based on photos and videos taken on-site, WhatsApp messages by Raniere and others, interviews with former members of his cult as well as with others who were witness to the goings-on, and more, the series describes in detail the horrifying psychopathic brutality of Raniere, specifically toward a group of women who were emotionally intimidated and blackmailed, sexually exploited, starved, locked up, and even hot-branded like animals with the initials of his name.

On the other end of the spectrum, a completely different type of narcissism that has positive aspects was labeled by Ronningstam (2005) as "extraordinary." As indicated by clinical evidence, narcissists are in many cases productive individuals with high standards who use their special talents to the benefit of society. Their characteristics are similar, but not identical, to those of the high-functioning exhibitionists described by Russ et al. (2008).

Narcissism may thus be expressed in various ways, depending to a large extent on the level of personality organization (i.e., moral awareness and values, the level of defense mechanisms, impulse control), which also bears on the type of narcissism – grandiose narcissism or covert/shy narcissism. But whatever the type or severity of narcissism or the level of personality organization, grandiosity – whether overt or covert, whether expressed at the high level of personality organization or at the lowest pathological level of personality organization – is invariably a key characteristic of the narcissist.

Yet grandiosity has another darker side. Once the actual or imagined narcissistic supply sustaining and reinforcing the grandiose sense of self is no longer available, the narcissist is hurled into the other extreme of the narcissistic experience, a devastating self-experience of vulnerability, imperfection, and inferiority. These two alternately dominant self-states – the grandiose self-state and the inferior self-state – are indicative of the narcissist's dissociative experience of the self, namely, the narcissist's split personality (Afek, 2018). In a sense, the clinical picture of distinct personality states presented in dissociative identity disorder is found in narcissistic personality disorder as well, as reflected in the presence of the two self-states that are dissociated on the experiential level. Thus, for instance, when the narcissist experiences himself as flawed and inferior, he still remembers his achievements or his inflated, omnipotent self-image, but his memory on the cognitive level seems to have no relevance for or effect on his negative experience of the self at that point. Similarly, when he experiences himself as superior and omnipotent, he is dissociated from his experience of the self as flawed and inferior. The sharp fluctuations between these two self-states reflect the narcissist's inability to develop a balanced and integrated sense of self. It should be emphasized, however, that unlike the case of dissociative identity disorder, the narcissist's dissociative experience of the self is not as extreme and does not involve defining features of the dissociative identity disorder such as discontinuity of identity, wherein one of the dissociative identities takes over and acts with the others unaware, or dissociative amnesia, manifested in gaps in memory of personal life events or everyday happenings, or multiplicity of dissociative identities.

The narcissistic supply may be cut off due to negative feedback at work, rejection by a romantic partner, unmet need for admiration, failure in the business arena, and so on. In many cases, the failures are subjectively perceived as such, but whether real or imagined, the ensuing collapse into an experience of the self as flawed and inferior triggers depression, anxiety, a feeling of emptiness, low self-esteem, lack of confidence in one's abilities, and, in severe cases, even suicidal thoughts. The duality of the narcissistic experience, fluctuating between inflated and deflated self-esteem, was aptly illustrated by Miller (1981) in her discussion of the gifted child:

> The collapse of self-esteem in a "grandiose" person will show clearly how precariously that self-esteem had been hanging in the air – "hanging from a balloon," a female patient once dreamed. That balloon flew up very high in a good wind but then suddenly got a hole and soon lay like a little rag on the ground. . . . For nothing genuine that could have given strength and support later on had even been developed.
>
> (p. 39)

The metaphor of the punctured balloon calls to mind the narcissistic display of grandiosity by Icarus, who, ignoring his limitations, ventured too high, too close to the sun, and fell to his death in the sea. The "Icarus complex"[1] is used to refer to the narcissistic character "fixated on Icarian pursuits of unattainable goals. These characters have 'peak and fall' experiences as they oscillate between periods of intense achievements . . . and flat periods of dissatisfaction, emptiness, depression" (Ronningstam, 2005, p. 9).

The sharp fluctuations between the two extreme poles of the narcissist's sense of self have been widely discussed in the recent literature (Diamond et al., 2013; Lingiardi & McWilliams, 2017; Pincus et al., 2014, among others). The issue is referred to in Section III of the DSM-5, although the lasting and enduring nature of the narcissist's dissociative experience of the self, that is, its characterization in terms of a split personality (Afek, 2018), is not discussed in the DSM-5. The frequency of the fluctuations in the narcissist's sense of self and their severity depend on the level of personality organization as well as on the presence of other personality traits. The lower the level of personality organization and the more prominent the presence of borderline personality traits, the more frequent and drastic the fluctuations between the grandiose self-state and the inferior self-state.

"I feel like I am worth nothing," one of my patients, a single businessman aged 40, once told me after losing in a virtual computer game played against anonymous participants. He felt so down that he shut himself up at home for several days, virtually crushed by his self-perception as an utter failure, unable to experientially recall his impressive achievements not only in the gaming arena but also and primarily in his thriving businesses, of which he used to boast with an inflated sense of self-importance. When in the grandiose self-state, feeling successful and thus superior to others, he would talk derogatorily about his friends. "Those losers, who have no real talent or ability, will have to work in menial jobs to make a living while I don't have to work another day in my life." On other occasions, when in the inferior self-state, he could think of nothing but his flaws, shortcomings, and failings compared with others, for instance, his failure to establish stable couple relationships and raise a family.

The narcissist's dissociative experience of the self accounts for his tireless efforts to sustain his illusory grandiose sense of self and show off his supremacy and superiority. After all, unless he can maintain an image of a perfect, superior, and omnipotent self, he is destined to collapse into the other extreme of the narcissistic experience, the devastating self-experience of vulnerability, imperfection, and inferiority. Narcissistic grandiosity is thus commonly seen as a pathological phenomenon and as a defense against deep-seated threatening mental content and disturbing emotions, such as fears of dependence, abandonment anxiety, depression, and feelings of imperfection or worthlessness (Afek, 2018; Bromberg, 2009; Diamond et al., 2022; Kernberg, 1975; Modell, 1975; Rosenfeld, 1964; Symington, 1993; McWilliams, 2011; Perry & Presniak, 2013).

Schizoidism

As part of the effort to maintain and sustain a sense of superiority, and hence invulnerability, the narcissist pictures himself as self-sufficient, as if he needs no one and as if anyone is easily replaceable. His self-sufficiency and avoidance of close, intimate relationships that involve emotional dependence are another facet of his narcissistic personality and, as suggested, a core feature of narcissism – termed in this context *schizoidism*.

Going back to the myth of Narcissus, it appears that along with his grandiosity, Narcissus displayed prominent schizoid characteristics. He was obsessively preoccupied with himself and his beauty, showed no real interest in others, and repulsed his many suitors, rejecting their love. However, close intimate relationships with a loving other are a fundamental innate need central to the human psyche, and the failure to acknowledge it is indicative of a defensive position. Indeed, as the ancient Greek myth suggests, Narcissus was desperately in need of love, and his apparent indifference and cold attitude toward others were merely a defensive posture. Thus, eventually, his deep-seated yearning for a close relationship and love culminated in his tragic end, when he fell madly in love with his own image, reflected in the water. Such a situation, where the other (in the case of Narcissus, his image reflected in the pool) is imaginary or inaccessible, provides a safe refuge for those who are unable to maintain close relationships with a real other. Typically, they fall in love with partners who live in a faraway country, are married, or have relationships with multiple partners.

While grandiosity has been discussed at length in the literature, the schizoid aspect of the narcissistic personality has been generally overlooked or only cursorily dealt with. This is true for the DSM-5, the *Psychodynamic Diagnostic Manual* (2nd ed.; PDM-2; Lingiardi & McWilliams, 2017), and the writings of Kohut, which are centered on the concept of narcissism. Still, schizoidism has been identified as a key feature of narcissism by various theorists, among them Kernberg (1975), Modell (1975), Volkan (1979), Symington (1993), Little (2006), and Perry and Presniak (2013). Symington is one of the prominent theorists who highlighted schizoidism as a core feature of narcissism. To illustrate the schizoid choice of fantasy over real-life relationships, Symington (1993) narrated the myth of Cassius, a young man who was lost in the outback and wandered for days in the wilderness, unable to find his way back home, until he chanced upon an enchanted paradise with fruit trees of various kinds, a sparkling freshwater stream flowing through, and a beautiful nymph who was at his service, ready to fulfill all his needs, playing enchanting music to entertain him, reading out engaging novels to amuse him, and sexually gratifying him. However, after about a year of blissful abandon, Cassius woke up one morning with feelings of restlessness, loneliness, and longing for a close relationship with a human being like him. Setting out in search of a human companion, he met a young woman named Miriam, who was rowing a boat in a river. She invited him to join her and have a baby with her, but that on one condition – the move to the other side of the bank was to be irreversible, the boat had to be burned, and there would be no way back to the dreamy wonderland he had been living in. Cassius hesitated and, reluctant to give up his piece of paradise, made a schizoid choice and rejected her offer. When after a while he regretted his choice, he discovered that it was too late. Miriam was already living with another man and raising their baby boy. In despair, Cassius drowned himself in the river.

The myth of Cassius is still relevant in our time and age. The contemporary Cassius is surfing the Internet, leading his life in the virtual space through his avatar, a successful, good-looking, adored hero whose needs are satisfied by other imaginary characters. Would he give up the virtual world in favor of real-life relationships along with their complexities, limitations, and emotional risks? Like Cassius, many today choose to remain entrenched in their make-believe virtual paradise, turning their back on the real world and on a close intimate relationship with a real other. However, as Symington (1993) observed, "the self is inherently relational . . . the core of narcissism is a hatred of the relational – a hatred of something that is inherent in our being" (p. 18). Symington traced this "hatred of the relational" to the traumatic denial of the innate infantile need for a life-giving object and the choice made already in infancy to turn away from the parental figure, described by Symington as the "lifegiver . . . the source of emotional life and . . . biological survival" (p. 39). While the attribution of a conscious choice to a child so early in his life seems implausible, it is argued, in line with Symington, that the rejection of the "lifegiver" – reflecting the schizoid aspect of the narcissistic personality – is at the core of narcissism and directly manifested in the self-sufficiency of the grandiose self, who needs no one.

Freud (1914/1957) addressed the schizoidism of the self-sufficient narcissist, although not labeling it as such, as a significant feature of the narcissistic phenomenon alongside grandiosity, observing that the secondary, pathological narcissistic process was characterized by the withdrawal of the libido from the external world into the ego – that is, the schizoid withdrawal from interpersonal relationships into an inner world. Freud described the phenomenon as displayed by narcissistic women, noting that "it is only themselves that such women love with an intensity comparable to that of the man's love for them. Nor does their need lie in the direction of loving, but of being loved; and the man who fulfils this condition is the one who finds favour with them" (p. 89).

Fairbairn (1952) discussed schizoidism without direct reference to narcissism. However, as noted by Kealy and Ogrodniczuk (2014) as well as by Symington (1993), Fairbairn's account of the schizoid personality corresponds to a large extent to the characterization of the narcissistic personality in contemporary literature. The same is true for the discussion of schizoidism by Guntrip (1968/1992). Elaborating on Fairbairn's conceptualization of schizoidism, Guntrip, who underwent analysis with Fairbairn and followed in his footsteps, highlighted the co-occurrence of grandiosity, which, as noted, is a core feature of narcissism, and avoidant schizoid characteristics – introversion, self-directed libido, and withdrawal into an inner world. Granting that Fairbairn's account of the schizoid personality closely matches the characterization of the narcissistic personality, his description of the psychodynamics of the schizoid personality would be applicable to the narcissistic personality as well. According to Fairbairn, the innate need for interpersonal relationships is the driving force around which the personality is organized. However, the schizoid, who is haunted by complex relationships with internal objects that are internalized representations of abusive or frustrating relationships in early childhood, gives up on close real-life interpersonal relationships. Recreating over and over again the negative relationships he experienced in his infancy, the schizoid is thus unable to establish meaningful close relationships with real people later on in his life, keeping aloof and self-centered, interacting with his internalized objects and no one else.

Kernberg (1975) maintained that narcissistic schizoidism, manifested in the avoidance of emotional dependence on the other, who is perceived as potentially hostile, was a key characteristic of the narcissistic personality:

> From the viewpoint of the patient's pathology, the advantage of a complete characterological "isolation" from any meaningful interpersonal relationship is hard to give up. These patients are able internally to withdraw from social life as effectively as the most severe schizoid character. And yet, they usually seem to be in the center of things, efficiently extracting "narcissistic supplies" while subtly protecting themselves from the painful experience of more meaningful emotional interactions.
>
> (p. 248)

The narcissist was variously described as withdrawing into a "glass bubble fantasy" (Volkan, 1979), a "cocoon" (Modell, 1975; Symington, 1993), or a "narcissistic envelope" (Symington, 1993) that served as an invisible protective wall separating him from the outside world. This self-protective schizoid glass bubble or cocoon, wherein the narcissist runs a kind of autarky, shields him from the risk of emotional intimacy with and rejection by the other, allowing him an illusion of perfection and self-sufficiency.

Clinical evidence supports these observations, showing that narcissists tend to avoid close intimate relationships and to the extent that they have any social relationships, these are essentially functional, no-strings-attached relationships where anyone is easily replaceable (Campbell & Baumeister, 2006; Carroll, 1987; Emmons, 1989). Bowlby (1988), who highlighted the fundamental centrality of emotional attachment in mental life, discussed the defensive avoidance of close intimate relationships – the anxious-avoidant attachment style, as he labeled it – which in severe cases could be diagnosed as narcissistic:

> A third pattern is that of the anxious avoidant attachment in which the individual has no confidence that, when he seeks care, he will be responded to helpfully but, on the contrary, expects to be rebuffed. When in marked degree such an individual attempts to live his life without the love and support of others, he tries to become emotionally self-sufficient and may later be diagnosed as narcissistic or as having a false self of the type described by Winnicott (1960).
>
> (pp. 124–125)

Studies in the realm of attachment theory provide further support for the observations regarding the narcissistic avoidance of close dependency relationships. Research findings point to the prevalence of the dismissive-avoidant attachment style among narcissists (Diamond et al., 2022), reflected in self-sufficiency and denial of the need for emotional support by the parental figure, as a child, or by a significant other, as an adult, even in situations of emotional distress. At the same time, an apparently contrasting attachment style, known as anxious attachment, which involves manifestations of dependence on the object of attachment rather than self-sufficiency coupled with indifference toward the other, was identified in narcissistic patients. The apparent contradiction may be explained by the two alternating self-states typical of the narcissist – the superior grandiose self-state and the vulnerable inferior self-state. When the grandiose narcissistic defenses collapse and the flawed vulnerable self emerges, the narcissist experiences an overwhelming need for the other and dependence on the other. It appears then that contrasting working models of attachment are internalized by the narcissist (Cain et al., 2008; Meyer & Pilkonis, 2011) – the more dominant and stable model of dismissive-avoidant attachment displayed when the narcissist is in the grandiose self-state, while the model of anxious attachment manifested when he collapses into the other extreme of the vulnerable inferior self-state. Fonagy (2001), among others, highlighted the dismissive-avoidant attachment style as characteristic of the narcissistic personality. In this context, Fonagy discussed the two opposite types described by Balint (1968) – the love-seeking and intensely dependent "ocnophil" and the aloof "dismissing philobat" who "dislikes attachments but loves the spaces between them" (Fonagy, 2001, p. 183), where he finds safe refuge from interpersonal relationships. Fonagy, who for years explored the relationship between attachment theory and psychoanalysis, looking for the points of correspondence between the two, further noted with reference to Balint's description of the philobat that it "is perhaps the clearest statement of the match between analytic accounts of narcissism and a detached – dismissing attachment pattern" (p. 95).

Empirical evidence indicates that the dismissive-avoidant attachment style is essentially defensive. Thus, during the Ainsworth Strange Situation assessment procedure, which assessed attachment security among infants, some infants left by their mother for a short while seemed to be indifferent and disinterested when the mother returned. However, contrary to appearances, they showed clear physiological measures of distress (Kealy & Ogrodniczuk, 2014), manifesting an insecure-avoidant pattern of attachment, as Ainsworth labeled it – their behavior in the reunion episodes considered the most useful indicator of attachment quality. Using the terminology of attachment theory, it may then be concluded that like any human being, the narcissist is in need of a close relationship with a significant other. However, adopting a defensive position, he pictures himself as self-sufficient, as if he needs no one, and rather than relying on the other, he relies on himself alone as a secure base (Holmes, 2001).

A., a patient of mine, a 27-year-old good-looking woman working as the VP of a high-tech company, sought psychotherapy due to panic attacks, which became all the more acute following the threat to fire her. Although she was appreciated as a talented and devoted worker, she found it difficult to accept authority and repeatedly clashed with her superiors. Likewise, she found it difficult to establish and maintain a stable couple relationship. She tended to choose as partners successful and impressive "alpha males," as she put it, acquiring a sense of self-value and a feeling of achievement from the relations with them. However, when she was spurned after a couple of months, as was often the case, she felt hurt, humiliated, and worthless. "I'm a failure. No one really wants me. What's wrong with me?" she wondered in pain. She feared that she would never find true love and would never manage to build a lasting couple relationship. Yet she never expressed sorrow or longing for the man who left her, with whom she had been madly in love not long before and whom she even hoped to marry. Once she met another alpha male, she seemed to undergo a drastic change of mood and felt great once again, forgetting all about her previous partner, as if he was erased from her mind. She almost never mentioned her ex-partners in the therapeutic sessions. She reminded me of the narcissistic women described by Reich (1953), who use men as mere replaceable objects, exploiting them to acquire a sense of self-worth and maintain their grandiose self in a narcissistic relationship devoid of any real emotional attachment – and hence, when coming to an end, it is without agony or grief over the separation.

Naturally, a close intimate relationship exposes the partners to the relationship to potential vulnerability, which the narcissist would do his best to avoid rather than deal with the involved distressing emotions, fears, and needs, which he denies for the most part, for instance, fear of losing control, mental pain, abandonment anxiety, longing, loneliness, the need for emotional intimacy, envy, or fear of rejection. The narcissist thus attempts to jump over the intimidating hurdle of an intimate relationship with the other by turning the other into an extension of the self or an object at his service, thereby securing control over the relationship and escaping susceptibility to the risks involved in the relationship. As shown in the following chapter, Freud, Winnicott, and Kohut failed to place due emphasis in their theories on the meaning of the loss of a significant other, a failure that reflects their narcissistic difficulty in acknowledging the unique, irreplaceable nature of close relationships with a significant other.

The narcissistic difficulty in establishing emotional intimacy with and dependence on the other is clearly demonstrated in the therapeutic setting with narcissistic patients, who adopt a detached and even belittling position with respect to the therapist. This defensive position shields the narcissistic patient from the risk of emotional dependence that is inherent in his relationship with the therapist (Rosenfeld, 1964). Thus, taking the position that he needs no one, the narcissist would do anything to avoid psychotherapy in the first place. When nevertheless he seeks psychotherapy, mostly due to a major crisis in his life, acute symptoms that trigger severe distress, or under the pressure of a spouse, he makes it a point to convey the message that the therapist has nothing to contribute to the therapeutic process. And even when experiencing acute mental stress, in most cases, the narcissistic patient refrains from seeking the therapist's emotional support, whether by asking for another weekly session, explicitly expressing his need for counseling, or in any other way. Furthermore, when sharing his painful experiences with the therapist, the narcissistic patient usually relates his woes in a detached, unemotional, or cynical manner and disdainfully rejects the therapist's counsel. It should be noted, though, that when the narcissistic patient collapses into the other extreme of the vulnerable, flawed, and inferior self-state, he may manifest his dependence on the therapist and need for the therapist's support.

The difficulty of acknowledging the otherness and separateness of the other

While narcissistic schizoidism is revealed in the context of close relationships with significant figures, the difficulty acknowledging the otherness and separateness of the other, which, as suggested, is another core feature of narcissism, is manifested in distant interpersonal relationships as well or even with regard to complete strangers (Akhtar, 2009; Benjamin, 1990; Bollas, 2000; Bromberg, 2009; Diamond et al., 2022; McDougall, 1985; Rosenfeld, 1964; Symington, 1993). The narcissist expects the other to adapt to his feelings and views and to serve as his extension to all intents and purposes, to the point of blurring the boundaries between the self and the other and obscuring the otherness and separateness of the other. Bollas (2000) enlarged on the narcissistic difficulty of acknowledging the otherness and separateness of the other:

> All will go fruitfully until such time as the other disagrees. It is not simply that the narcissist finds differences with the self difficult to take, but difference in itself is hard to bear. Indeed, the narcissist's strategy is largely aimed at oblating differences between self and other, seeking relations with common objects around which idealisation may occur.
>
> (p. 8)

In this context, Bollas (2000) further noted that the narcissist seeks "to take refuge in a semi-fortified Arcadian world of self-objects" (p. 9). It should be noted, however, that it is not simply "oblating differences between self and other" (p. 8), as Bollas put it, that the narcissist is seeking. In fact, the narcissist attempts to obliterate the uniqueness of the other rather than his own perceived distinctiveness. He perceives his own otherness and distinctiveness as reflecting a superior uniqueness, which all others should acknowledge, admire, and conform to. Thus, a narcissistic CEO would expect his subordinates to categorically agree with him, or else they could be seen as harboring malicious thoughts about him and suffer his wrath.

The narcissistic aspiration for "ideal" flawless relationships of blind compliance is similarly evident in the arena of couple interactions, where almost total spousal conformity is expected. The narcissist may describe such relationships as symbiotic. However, rather than a mutually beneficial alliance, it is a one-way relationship, where the narcissist's way of life, his beliefs, positions, and wishes in various areas (parenting, friends, politics, etc.) prevail, leaving no room for a free dialogue between two separate persons. A patient of mine once told me that he offered his wife to open up their relationship. Since she did not explicitly veto the option, he assumed that the arrangement was commonly agreed by them and went on to engage in extramarital affairs. The truth was that she was afraid of entering into an ongoing conflict with him that would inevitably lead to separation and thus refrained from openly confronting him. Deep inside, she was enraged and envious. Her hard feelings were coupled with abandonment anxiety, which she found difficult to admit. Partners like her who tend to assimilate, so to speak, into the narcissistic personality of their mate are often characterized by borderline personality traits, including uncertainty about self-worth and unstable, vaguely defined self-identity. They are easily influenced by others, all the more so by charismatic figures, as narcissists often are. They thus tend to adopt the views and positions of their narcissistic partner and in exchange gain a positive or even a loving attitude.

The otherness of the other is either ignored by the narcissist or met with suspicion, mistrust, or a condescending attitude and, in some cases, triggers outright hostility. Such narcissistic attitudes may be manifested in the public arena, in the marginalization and exclusion of minority populations, nonconforming groups, or people with unorthodox views or lifestyles, as well as in interpersonal relationships that are characterized by a persistent narcissistic pattern of disdain of or antagonism toward the other, or utter disregard of the other and the otherness of the other.

O., a 40-year-old patient of mine, although not diagnosed as psychotic, entertained an enduring image of himself as a unique human being, the only being of significance in the world, the protagonist of a movie revolving around his life, where all others were mere background actors designed to serve him. The false reality O. lived in is reminiscent, in a sense, of *The Truman Show*. However, unlike the lead character in the thought-provoking film bearing his name, who was unaware that his entire life was a reality TV show taking place on a movie set, where he was involuntarily and unknowingly filmed around the clock, O. was convinced that he was the hero in his own scripted show of his life, an illusion that subsided with time although it has never completely disappeared. Similar cases of two patients, each of whom envisioned himself in his childhood as the only human being on Earth, were reported by Symington (1993).

The deep-rooted narcissistic need to deny the existence of the other as a separate entity was less dramatically displayed in the case of another patient of mine. D., a 55-year-old man, showed a consistent behavior pattern in social settings of haughty disregard of the others. He used to dominate the conversation, talking nonstop, loudly and theatrically, telling jokes, recounting his adventurous travels around the world, discussing the books he read, the movies he watched, and the philosophical teachings of the gurus he met during his trips to the East. He hardly let anyone get a word in. As it emerged during therapy, he felt that if his voice was not exclusively heard, no one would notice him and his presence would be erased. He found it difficult to consider the middle option that would allow room for his own voice as well as for that of the others. His difficulty acknowledging the presence of and allowing room for the other was reflected in his relationship with his wife as well. In one of the sessions, he told me that while working in the garden with his wife during the weekend, he repeatedly criticized her, complaining that she was too slow, carelessly pruned the branches, or thoughtlessly arranged the backyard toolshed. When I asked him how he thought she experienced the situation, he seemed unable to relate to her feelings. Instead, he came up with all sorts of explanations for her apparent misperformance. "The garden at her parents' place is untended . . . she has no awareness of the way a garden should be cultivated . . . no one has taught her how to work efficiently." When I asked him once again to try and think how she felt about the situation, to try and see it from her point of view, carefully confronting him with her otherness and separateness (using a strategy that, I believe, enables self-development and is conducive to the therapeutic process), he was thrown off balance. He looked confused and nervous (although on other occasions, when confronted with challenging issues, his reaction was quite different). He tried to change the topic, smiling uneasily. Evidently, he found it difficult to cope with the request to acknowledge the presence of his wife as a separate human being with feelings, thoughts, and wishes of her own that were not necessarily in agreement with the way he saw her – as a separate object, albeit reduced and weakened, without a significant subjective existence of her own.

The ability to acknowledge the otherness of the other as a separate human being with sensations, emotions, volition, and thoughts of his own was highlighted by Benjamin (1990) as indicative of personality maturity and as enabling enjoyable interpersonal relationships. According to Benjamin, the recognition of the other as such would counterbalance the omnipotent narcissistic experience of exclusivity and domination over the other:

> Our psychic makeup is such that we are torn between omnipotence, the illusion of control, on the one hand, and the wish for contact with the different, the external, the not-me, on the other. The "solution" – insofar as we may speak of one – to this conflict is that . . . we become dialecticians who can hold such opposites in tension . . . so we can posit an inherent conflict in intersubjective life between eros and narcissism, recognition and omnipotence. The tension that we ideally imagine between these continually breaks down and has to be accomplished over and over.
>
> (p. 202)

Yet it seems that the narcissist is trapped in a rigid omnipotent position that rules out movement toward mutual recognition between two subjects. At times, his overt behavior may seem to be at odds with his ingrained narcissistic omnipotence. Thus, the narcissist may momentarily appear to ignore his own needs, wishes, and subjectivity and to make room for the other in order to please and impress the other and gain his admiration. In longer-term relationships, the narcissist may assume the role of the martyr and sacrifice his needs and wishes in exchange for an adoring and idolizing attitude on the part of the other, thus securing the dependence of the other while maintaining and enhancing his own omnipotent experience of grandiosity.

The typical narcissistic denial of the separate presence of the other is clearly manifested in the psychotherapeutic setting, where the therapist serves as a significant figure for the patient. The narcissistic patient may behave as if the therapist is invisible and there is no one else in the room, thus erecting a defensive wall between him and the therapist, whose separate presence threatens him. B., a 25-year-old patient of mine, made it clear right at the outset that she intended to take the starring role. "I am not interested in you, and do me a favor, don't tell me anything about you. It would just make things more difficult. As far as I'm concerned, you better be like the flowerpot in the corner of the room or the picture on the wall, unobtrusively present, and that's it."

McDougall (1985) illustrated the difficulty of the narcissistic patient in acknowledging the separate presence of the therapist through the experience of one of her patients who was irritated by the tone of her voice that "penetrated her like foreign bodies which [she had] to take time to digest" (p. 231). As McDougall noted, her patient was actually troubled to find that they were two separate persons. As a therapist, I have realized that while non-narcissistic patients often notice and occasionally react to changes in my appearance, mood, or health (e.g., a sudden hoarseness of voice, a new haircut, or unusually high spirits) or show interest in me in other ways, narcissistic patients behave as if I am not there. They see me merely in terms of my function as a therapist, ignoring my presence as a separate human being with a life of my own.

Kohut, for his part, believed that the therapist should adopt an empathetic vantage point and attune himself as far as possible to the patient while playing down his own otherness and separateness. As shown in the next chapter, Kohut himself displayed narcissistic personality traits and could thus identify with the need of his narcissistic patients to deny and reject the otherness and separateness of the therapist. However, as suggested, confronting the narcissistic patient with the otherness and separateness of the therapist is essential to the therapeutic process. It should be borne in mind that the narcissist finds it difficult to accept the fact that the other, the therapist in this case, has something of value to offer him, as it undermines his illusion of perfection. Thus, paradoxically, while seeking expert counseling, the narcissistic patient does his best to show that he has no need for the therapist or his counsel.

Bach (1985) addressed the issue from the analyst's perspective:

> Analysts who work with narcissistic patients complain frequently on the difficulty they experience in "getting through" to the patient and "making themselves heard," or, with growing irritation, they speak of

> "making a dent" in the patient or "cracking the narcissistic shell." They sometimes develop an intense feeling of frustration about the impermanence of even their effective interpretations and compare it with talking into the wind or writing on the sand, only to have one's words effaced moments later by the waves.
>
> (p. 3)

Rosenfeld (1971) discussed the dynamics of the therapeutic process with the focus on the entrenched position of the narcissistic patient:

> In my previous work on narcissism (1964) I stressed the projective and introjective identification of self and object (fusion of self and object) in narcissistic states, which act as a defense against any recognition of separateness between the self and objects. Awareness of separation immediately leads to feelings of dependence on an object and therefore to inevitable frustrations. However, dependence also stimulates envy, when the goodness of the object is recognized. Aggressiveness towards objects therefore seems inevitable in giving up the narcissistic position and it appears that the strength and persistence of omnipotent narcissistic object relations is closely related to the strength of the envious destructive impulses.
>
> (p. 172)

It may thus be concluded that grandiosity, schizoidism, and the difficulty acknowledging the otherness and separateness of the other are the three core features and diagnostic hallmarks of the narcissistic personality. However, the picture is far more complex and multifaceted than it may appear. For one thing, it should be noted that these core features are evaluated along a continuum of severity, from the mild to the acute, rather than in terms of absolute values – present or absent. Thus, for instance, narcissists with acute schizoidism are unable to establish and maintain emotionally close interpersonal relationships, while in milder cases, close intimate relationships may be established, generally, with a few family members. The more severe the personality pathology, the more prominent the presence of the core features of narcissism, and vice versa.

The grandiose position of the narcissist, his denial of the innate need for a close intimate relationship with a significant other, and his difficulty seeing the therapist as a separate human being constitute a huge challenge for the therapist, requiring maturity, professional confidence, and perseverance on his part. Of course, as noted, narcissistic patients may differ in various ways. They may be characterized by varying severity levels of pathology as well as by the various types of narcissism. They may display arrogant grandiosity or be of the vulnerable shy type. The latter tend to be less aggressive and less derogatory and are thus less challenging for the therapist. The level of personality organization is another aspect that comes into play in this context.

Naturally, the higher the level of personality organization, the less stressful the therapeutic process. Characterizations aside, each patient has a unique personality and is a world in himself and should be regarded as such.

The following clinical case illustrates the way in which each of the core features of narcissism is manifested in the narcissistic personality.

N., a good-looking 34-year-old musician with a slim build and average height, sought psychotherapy in a depressive, suicidal state of mind, urged by one of his acquaintances to apply for professional help. He appeared to be shy and somewhat childish, with a mysterious charm about him. He described himself as a loner, living by himself in a rented apartment in a vibrant big city, where he used to shut himself up for hours on end, sleeping or playing the piano. He regularly smoked weed to bolster his mood. He felt that he could not do without it, in particular, when getting up in the morning. N. was still struggling to make ends meet, relying on occasional jobs, mostly as a musician, playing with music groups, teaching music, and so on. However, he never kept any job for too long and had to fall back on the financial support of his parents, who were living overseas. His outbursts of rage, provoked by even the slightest criticism, which was perceived by him as an attack on him personally, were the main reason for his erratic job record. While he was invariably welcomed by new band mates as a highly skilled performer and even gained their affection thanks to his personal charm and usually pleasant demeanor, sooner or later he would quit in anger due to differences of opinion over the band's playing style or the way he played a certain piece of music. He seemed unable to accept disagreement with his musical taste and preferences or to acknowledge the fact that others too could have something to contribute and that there was room for a diversity of tastes and styles, whether in music or in any other area. Following such incidents, N., clearly upset, used to deride his ex-band members, indignantly noting that compared with him, "those guys" were way under par, "amateurs who understand nothing about music" and thus unworthy of his time and efforts. While generally seen as gentle and unassuming, his underlying condescending attitude toward others became apparent when he felt criticized, threatened, or otherwise vulnerable and inferior. Thus, for instance, he talked contemptuously about acquaintances of his, "those shallow and spineless bourgeois couples" who were stuck in a rut and only interested in getting established financially. On other, less frequent occasions, his grandiosity was revealed when he shared with me his daydreams about monumental success on the most prestigious stages in the world. His grandiose fantasies of international acclaim were similarly sparked by delighted audiences following especially successful performances or by positive feedback from esteemed performers. However, once he experienced a setback, whether real or imaginary, he was thrown back into the other extreme of vulnerability and inferiority, feeling a complete failure.

As a child, N. was considered a prodigy. His good looks landed him a lucrative contract as the star of a commercial for a popular kids candy, by which his parents made a lot of money. One of his formative childhood memories was the scorn on the part of his school mates, who ridiculed him for not being enough of a "boy" with real interest in football, combat computer games, or other competitive and aggressive games typically played by boys. Instead, N. used to spend hours playing the piano, creating intricate origami models, or painting in watercolors. He felt that his artistic interests and "effeminate" gentle manner deeply disappointed his father. His mother was a career woman with too little time for her children, and both parents were often absent due to their frequent work trips abroad.

N. was confused about his sexual identity. He had sexual relationships with both women and men, who fell desperately in love with him, captivated by his beauty and charm. However, he experienced their love as suffocating and furiously rejected them when they sought a more meaningful emotional intimacy. He never showed empathy for any of them and never expressed guilt for hurting them or wish to see them. His love affairs were short-lived, lasting no more than several months, and his few social relationships were essentially functional and superficial. In family gatherings N. felt ill at ease, as if critically examined under a magnifying glass. And even his relationships with his close family – his parents, his brother, and his three sisters – were cold and distant. They disapproved of his way of life and were disappointed at his failure to establish a stable couple relationship and to secure financial independence. No wonder then that he hardly, if ever, discussed his life with them.

N. was equally reticent in the therapeutic setting. He often missed sessions, his excuse being that he simply forgot all about it, and when he did show up, he hardly talked and gave the impression of being emotionally remote and unavailable. Yet, on the whole, my therapeutic relationship with him was quite good. I liked him and was enchanted by his mysterious charm. I noticed though that, unlike my habit with other patients, I rarely thought about him in between sessions. It could be his own aloofness that gave rise to the feeling of detachment.

It appears then that N. was the typical vulnerable, shy narcissist – his covert sense of grandiosity revealed in his fantasies about monumental success and international acclaim and in his refusal to accept anything less than that. As he himself admitted, nothing less than grandiose success could satisfy him, and as long as he did not achieve it, he considered himself a total failure. The schizoid core of his personality was manifested in his denial of his deep-seated need for emotional intimacy, reflected in his avoidance of any meaningful close relationship as well as in his detached attitude in the therapeutic setting. His difficulty acknowledging the otherness and separateness of the other and to accept or even consider the views and preferences of the other was evident in his relations and conflicts with band mates as well as in his disdainful comments on the lifestyle and values of others.

As to the therapeutic implications, the diagnosis of these core features of narcissism calls for specific therapeutic foci beyond the more general comprehensive process. Specifically, an effective therapeutic approach that addresses all facets of the narcissistic personality and promotes personality integration should be adopted (Afek, 2018). Along with the integration of the two dissociated states of the self, the grandiose and inferior self-states, an attempt should be made to get through the narcissistic schizoid shell and encourage the patient to acknowledge his innate, albeit denied need for emotional intimacy. At the same time, exercising due caution, the patient should be confronted with the otherness and separateness of the other, both in the therapeutic setting and with reference to his interpersonal relationships outside the therapeutic setting.

Is there healthy narcissism?

In contrast to the view of narcissism as pathological and defensive, Kohut perceived narcissism as a natural and healthy phenomenon that is not defensive and that may even reflect highly developed mental abilities. Kohut's theory, which is centered on the phenomenon of narcissism, is of special interest in this context as it has vastly influenced psychoanalysis, in general, and the professional discourse and practice, in particular. According to Kohut (1966), the view of narcissism as pathological originates in prejudice and cultural bias:

> Although in theoretical discussions it will usually not be disputed that narcissism, the libidinal investment of the self, is per se neither pathological nor obnoxious, there exists an understandable tendency to look at it with a negatively toned evaluation as soon as the field of theory is left. Where such a prejudice exists, it is undoubtedly based on a comparison between narcissism and object love, and is justified by the assertion that it is the more primitive and the less adaptive of the two forms of libido distribution. I believe, however, that these views do not stem primarily from an objective assessment either of the developmental position or of the adaptive value of narcissism, but that they are due to the improper intrusion of the altruistic value system of Western civilization.
>
> (p. 243)

In fact, as Kohut argued, a primary, archaic, primitive form of narcissism is transformed "into more highly differentiated, new psychological configurations" (p. 257) – this, provided the basic narcissistic needs are fulfilled in early childhood or in the course of psychoanalytic therapy. Narcissistic energies are thus transformed into more highly developed forms such as empathy, wisdom, creativity, humor, and the capacity to acknowledge the finiteness of individual existence. With reference to the relationship between creativity (and productivity) and narcissistic energy, Kohut (1978) noted:

> No doubt all creative and productive work depends on the employment of both grandiose *and* idealizing narcissistic energies, but I think that truly original thought, i.e., creativity, is energized predominantly

> from the grandiose self, while the work of more tradition-bound scientific and artistic activities, i.e., productivity, is performed with idealizing cathexes.
>
> (p. 801)

In other words, according to Kohut, creativity and the other more highly developed psychological configurations, or abilities, are driven by and draw strength from narcissistic energy, which is thus seen as a resource for mental health – in stark contrast to the view of narcissism as a pathological phenomenon. The conceptual ambiguity surrounding Kohut's proposed model of narcissism is discussed at length in my critique of Kohut's theory of self psychology (Afek, 2019). In a nutshell, it is unclear what Kohut meant when talking about narcissism – was it narcissism as a specific personality structure with a vertical split separating the two parts of the self, or narcissism as the phenomenon of a fragile and disintegrated self, or perhaps narcissism as the complex of phenomena related to the self and the processes that shape the self? There seems to be no clear-cut distinction in his theory between the concept of narcissism and the concept of the self. The conceptual ambiguity surrounding narcissism is not unique to Kohut. Over the years, the concept of narcissism has been variously perceived and interpreted in the literature (Cain et al., 2008; Kealy & Ogrodniczuk, 2014) and in the absence of a commonly agreed definition, there is still much confusion about the issue.

To discuss the question of whether there is healthy narcissism, we should first distinguish between narcissism as a phenomenon that is reflected in various ways and narcissism as manifested in the narcissistic personality, which is characterized by specific, well-defined and stable traits. Narcissism may be associated with various normative phenomena, for instance, the natural need to demonstrate special abilities, to achieve great success, or to win the admiration of others, or the common tendency to indulge in unrealistic fantasies or to entertain a sense of entitlement. The same holds true for occasional ups and downs in self-esteem, natural preoccupation with self-esteem, uncharacteristic outbursts of rage triggered by personal insults, atypical expression of arrogance, and so on. Commonly displayed in varying degrees by each and every one of us, all these may be seen as normal manifestations of narcissism. Thus, for instance, Mitchell (1986) saw the illusory omnipotent aspect of narcissism as healthy and normal and as stimulating curiosity, liveliness, and playfulness, this, in contrast to pathological narcissism, which is expressed in a rigid, obsessive, and addictive pattern of self-aggrandization and in clear preference for relationships that mirror the grandiose image of the self. Unlike the natural and normal universal narcissistic phenomena, the rigid patterns of behavior and relationships that Mitchell referred to actually reflect, as argued here, rigid and stable narcissistic personality traits. The discussion then revolves around the question of whether normal and healthy aspects of narcissism may be found in individuals with narcissistic personality traits that are broadly expressed in distinctive behavior patterns, subjective experience, and specific individual psychodynamics.

The ambiguity surrounding Kohut's model of narcissism and the diverse phenomena he considered narcissistic aside, judging by the clinical cases described in his writings, some of his patients would have no doubt been diagnosed with narcissistic personality disorder under the current diagnostic criteria. Yet at variance with most theorists (Kernberg, Modell, and Symington, among others), Kohut did not see the narcissistic personality as pathological. He ascribed the unregulated behavior displayed by his patients to unfulfilled needs in early childhood and maintained that a significant improvement toward more regulated behavior, personal vitality, and enhanced creativity could be achieved by means of psychoanalysis that would respond to the patient's narcissistic needs through selfobject transference in the context of the therapeutic relationship.

As noted, the majority of theorists are of the opinion that narcissism is essentially pathological. Thus, for instance, Symington (1993) explicitly stated that there could be no healthy narcissism since, by definition, narcissism was an expression of hate of parts of the self, which he traced back to the rejection of the "lifegiver." In this context, Symington noted, "Narcissism is nearly always the product of a trauma. The whole narcissistic way of functioning, the grandiosity and the disowning of parts of the self, is a defensive procedure" (p. 73).

The relevant question at the focus of the discussion can thus be rephrased as follows: Can we find normal and healthy aspects of narcissism in individuals who are diagnosed with personality pathology on one level or another? The answer depends on the level of personality organization, which is indicative of the level of pathology and, at the same time, may point to normal and even highly developed mental abilities in certain areas. The level of personality organization is evaluated along a continuum, from the lowest pathological level, through the borderline level and neurotic level, to the high, mature level of personality organization. It is determined based on relatively stable mental abilities, such as the ability to perceive and express various emotions, the ability to establish mutual close relationships, the ability to mentalize, and moral awareness and values, whether highly developed or pathological (Lingiardi & McWilliams, 2017). According to Kernberg (Diamond et al., 2022), the pathological grandiose self, which is a defensive personality structure, is manifest on all levels of personality organization. However, individuals with a high level of personality organization often display personal charm and stability in most areas of life and under most circumstances, unless they feel criticized or under a threat to their self-worth, in which case they show hostility and find it difficult to hold a dialogue. They generally maintain relatively stable and fulfilling, even though somewhat superficial, interpersonal and couple relationships, and for the most part, they are not aggressive. They resemble to a large extent the narcissists labeled by Ronningstam (2005) as "extraordinary" – described by her, although without direct reference to the level of personality organization, as creative, high achievers with an exceptionally high self-worth. In many cases they are charismatic leaders who translate ideas, ideals, and high goals into actual achievements, thus contributing to the benefit of society. Likewise, Russ et al. (2008) identified a subtype of narcissistic personality disorder labeled as high-functioning/exhibitionistic. Such individuals have significant psychological strengths, show good adaptive functioning and less psychiatric comorbidity, and are highly motivated, achievement oriented, and attention seeking grandstanders.

Miller (1981) described narcissists who are less aggressive than those commonly characterized as narcissists, who show sensitivity and empathy for others, and who tend to please the others and fulfill their needs while repressing their own. Her description fits the characterization of narcissists with a high level of personality organization, although Miller did not refer to them as such. As noted by Miller, psychoanalysts commonly display similar narcissistic characteristics:

> It is often said that psychoanalysts suffer from a narcissistic disturbance. The purpose of my presentation so far has been to clarify the extent to which this can be confirmed, not only inductively based on experience, but also deductively from the type of talent that is needed by an analyst. His sensibility, his empathy, his intense and differentiated emotional responsiveness, and his unusually powerful "antennae" seem to predestine him as a child to be used – if not misused – by people with intense narcissistic needs.
>
> (p. 22)

It can then be said that the lower the level of personality organization (specifically at the borderline and low levels of personality organization), the more socially destructive and self-destructive the narcissistic behavior, the more unstable and exploitative and the less empathetic the relationships the narcissist is involved in, the more difficult it is to keep any job for too long, the sharper and more frequent the fluctuations in the sense of self, and the less intact the reality testing. At the bottom of the scale, narcissism of the type labeled by Kernberg (2007) as malignant is displayed by psychopathic and sadistic narcissists, like Keith Raniere, the charismatic cult leader who exploited his followers to satisfy his own needs and desires.

At the same time, the higher the level of personality organization, the less pathological the narcissism and the more constructive its manifestations, as affecting the individual as well as the society he lives in. The narcissistic personality thus evidently has healthy aspects, especially, although not only at the higher levels of personality organization. The sense of grandiosity shared by all narcissists may serve as a powerful engine for achievement. Driven by self-confidence, boundless optimism, and high motivation, and setting high goals, narcissists have been visionary and courageous trailblazers, as shown throughout history in various areas of human endeavor – in the arts, in technology, and in social, political, and military leadership. In the business arena, too, larger-than-life narcissistic leaders have taken center stage (Maccoby, 2004), channeling their creativity and inventiveness to the benefit of their companies (Smith & Webster, 2018).

I believe that even narcissists with borderline personality organization may aspire to great achievements and, in some cases, manage to accomplish their goals thanks to their strong need and relentless efforts to demonstrate their abilities and unique contribution – this, in contrast to individuals with borderline personality traits, who lack focus in life and feel confused and in chaos. The narcissistic personality is less amorphous and more cohesive as it is organized around specific needs and goals that are of the utmost importance to the narcissist – first and foremost the need to maintain and flaunt his superiority. It thus allows relative stability, the achievement of goals, satisfaction and pride in oneself, and social recognition, thereby supporting and enhancing mental health (albeit at the cost of impoverishing the personality). It may explain why Blatt (2008) saw the narcissists as characterized by a more mature personality, as expressed inter alia in the use of more mature defense mechanisms, compared with others classified as introjective (the obsessives and the paranoids).

In conclusion, it is argued here and commonly held that narcissism is basically pathological. The narcissistic personality structure serves as a pathological defense against painful early childhood traumas. Yet at the higher levels of personality organization, the healthy aspects of the narcissistic personality come into play, and narcissism may be harnessed for the good of society and to the benefit of the individual himself.

Note

1 As noted by Ronningstam (2005, p. 9), "The 'Icarus complex' was identified by Murray (1955) in a phallic-narcissistic character."

References

Afek, O. (2018). The split narcissist: The grandiose self versus the inferior self. *Psychoanalytic Psychology, 35*(2), 231–236. https://doi.org/10.1037/pap0000161

Afek, O. (2019). Reflections on Kohut's theory of self psychology and pathological narcissism – Limitations and concerns. *Psychoanalytic Psychology, 36*(2), 166–172. https://doi.org/10.1037/pap0000201

Akhtar, S. (2009). Love, sex, and marriage in the setting of pathological narcissism. *Psychiatric Annals, 39*(4), 185–191.

American Psychiatric Association, DSM-5 Task Force. (2013). *Diagnostic and statistical manual of mental disorders. DSM-5*™ (5th ed.). American Psychiatric Publishing. https://doi.org/10.1176/appi.books.9780890425596

Bach, S. (1985). *Narcissistic states and the therapeutic process*. Jason Aronson.

Balint, M. (1968). *The basic fault: Therapeutic aspects of regression*. Routledge.

Benjamin, J. (1990). Recognition and destruction: An outline of intersubjectivity. In S. A. Mitchell & L. Aron (Eds.), *Relational psychoanalysis: The emergence of a tradition* (pp. 181–210). Routledge.

Blatt, S. J. (2008). *Polarities of experience: Relatedness and self-definition in personality development, psychopathology, and the therapeutic process*. American Psychological Association.

Bollas, C. (2000). *Hysteria*. Routledge.
Bowlby, J. (1988). *A secure base: Parent-child attachment and healthy human development*. Basic Books.
Bromberg, P. M. (2009). Discussion of Robert Grossmark's case of Pamela. *Psychoanalytic Dialogues, 19*(1), 31–38. https://doi.org/10.1080/10481880802634644
Cain, N. M., Pincus, A. L., & Ansell, E. B. (2008). Narcissism at the crossroads: Phenotypic description of pathological narcissism across clinical theory, social/personality psychology, and psychiatric diagnosis. *Clinical Psychology Review, 28*(4), 638–656. https://doi.org/10.1016/j.cpr.2007.09.006
Caligor, E. (2013). Narcissism in the psychodynamic diagnostic manual. In J. S. Ogrodniczuk (Ed.), *Understanding and treating narcissistic personality disorder* (pp. 235–252). American Psychological Association.
Campbell, W. K., & Baumeister, R. F. (2006). Narcissistic personality disorder. In J. E. Fisher & W. T. O'Donohue (Eds.), *Practitioner's guide to evidence-based psychotherapy* (pp. 423–431). Springer.
Carroll, L. (1987). A study of narcissism, affiliation, intimacy, and power motives among students in business administration. *Psychological Reports, 61*(2), 355–358. https://doi.org/10.2466/pr0.1987.61.2.355
Diamond, D., Yeomans, F. E., Stern, B. L., & Kernberg, O. F. (2022). *Treating pathological narcissism with transference-focused psychotherapy*. The Guilford Press.
Diamond, D., Yeomans, F. E., Stern, B., Levy, K. N., Hörz, S., Doering, S., & Clarkin, J. F. (2013). Transference focused psychotherapy for patients with comorbid narcissistic and borderline personality disorder. *Psychoanalytic Inquiry, 33*(6), 527–551. http://dx.doi.org/10.1080/07351690.2013.815087
Emmons, R. A. (1989). Exploring the relations between motives and traits: The case of narcissism. In D. M. Buss & N. Cantor (Eds.), *Personality psychology: Recent trends and emerging directions* (pp. 32–44). Springer.
Fairbairn, W. R. D. (1952). *Psychoanalytic studies of the personality*. Routledge.
Fonagy, P. (2001). *Attachment theory and psychoanalysis*. Other Press. (Original work published 1952)
Freud, S. (1957a). *On narcissism: An introduction* (J. Strachey, Ed. & Trans., Standard Edition, Vol. 14, 1914–1916, pp. 73–102). Hogarth Press. (Original work published 1914)
Freud, S. (1957b). *Some character-types met with in psycho-analytic work* (J. Strachey, Ed. & Trans., Standard Edition, Vol. 14, 1914–1916, pp. 309–333). Hogarth Press. (Original work published 1916)
Gabbard, G. O. (1989). Two subtypes of narcissistic personality disorder. *Bulletin of the Menninger Clinic, 53*(6), 527–532.
Guntrip, H. (1992). *Schizoid phenomena, object relations and the self*. Karnac Books. https://read.amazon.com/?asin=B005RX17FW&ref_=kwl_kr_iv_rec_15 (Original work published 1968)
Holmes, J. (2001). *Narcissism: Ideas in psychoanalysis*. Icon Books.
Horney, K. (2000). *New ways in psychoanalysis*. W. W. Norton. (Original work published 1939)
Kealy, D., & Ogrodniczuk, J. S. (2014). Pathological narcissism and the obstruction of love. *Psychodynamic Psychiatry, 42*(1), 101–119. http://dx.doi.org/10.1521/pdps.2014.42.1.101
Kernberg, O. F. (1975). *Borderline conditions and pathological narcissism*. Rowman & Littlefield. https://read.amazon.com/?asin=B00BZAMWA0&ref_=kwl_kr_iv_rec_23
Kernberg, O. F. (2007). The almost untreatable narcissistic patient. *Journal of the American Psychoanalytic Association, 55*(2), 503–539.
Kohut, H. (1966). Forms and transformations of narcissism. *Journal of the American Psychoanalytic Association, 14*(2), 243–272. https://doi.org/10.1177/000306516601400201

Kohut, H. (1978). *The search for the self: Selected writings of Heinz Kohut: 1950–1978. Vol. 2*. (P. H. Ornstein, Ed.). International Universities Press.
Lingiardi, V., & McWilliams, N. (Eds.). (2017). *Psychodynamic diagnostic manual: PDM-2* (2nd ed.). The Guilford Press.
Little, R. (2006). Treatment considerations when working with pathological narcissism. *Transactional Analysis Journal, 36*(4), 303–317.
Maccoby, M. (2004). Narcissistic leaders: The incredible pros, the inevitable cons. In A. Hooper (Ed.), *Leadership perspectives* (pp. 31–39). Routledge.
Masterson, J. F. (2013). *The narcissistic and borderline disorders: An integrated developmental approach*. Routledge. (Original work published 1981)
McDougall, J. (1985). *Theaters of the mind: Illusion and truth on the psychoanalytic stage*. Basic Books.
McWilliams, N. (2011). *Psychoanalytic diagnosis: Understanding personality structure in the clinical process* (2nd ed.). Guilford Press.
Meyer, B., & Pilkonis, P. A. (2011). Attachment theory and narcissistic personality disorder. In W. K. Campbell & J. D. Miller (Eds.), *The handbook of narcissism and narcissistic personality disorder: Theoretical approaches, empirical findings, and treatments* (pp. 434–444). John Wiley & Sons.
Miller, A. (1981). *The drama of the gifted child: The search for the true self* (R. Ward, Trans.). Basic Books.
Mitchell, S. A. (1986). The wings of Icarus: Illusion and the problem of narcissism. *Contemporary Psychoanalysis, 22*(1), 107–132. https://doi.org/10.1080/00107530.1986.10746118
Modell, A. H. (1975). A narcissistic defence against affects and the illusion of self-sufficiency. *The International Journal of Psychoanalysis, 56*(3), 275–282.
Morf, C. C. (2006). Personality reflected in a coherent idiosyncratic interplay of intra- and interpersonal self-regulatory. *Journal of Personality, 74*(6), 1527–1556.
Morf, C. C., & Rhodewalt, F. (2001). Unraveling the paradoxes of narcissism: A dynamic self-regulatory processing model. *Psychological Inquiry, 12*(4), 177–196.
Perry, J. C., & Presniak, M. D. (2013). Conflicts and defenses in narcissistic personality disorder. In J. S. Ogrodniczuk (Ed.), *Understanding and treating pathological narcissism* (pp. 147–166). American Psychological Association.
Pincus, A. L., Cain, N. M., & Wright, A. G. C. (2014). Narcissistic grandiosity and narcissistic vulnerability in psychotherapy. *Personality Disorders: Theory, Research, and Treatment, 5*(4), 439–443. https://doi.org/10.1037/per0000031
Reich, A. (1953). Narcissistic object choice in women. *Journal of the American Psychoanalytic Association, 1*(1), 22–44. https://doi.org/10.1177/000306515300100103
Ronningstam, E. (2005). *Identifying and understanding the narcissistic personality*. Oxford University Press.
Ronningstam, E., & Gunderson, J. G. (1990). Identifying criteria for narcissistic personality disorder. *The American Journal of Psychiatry, 147*(7), 918–922. https://doi.org/10.1176/ajp.147.7.918
Rosenfeld, H. (1964). On the psychopathology of narcissism: A clinical approach. *The International Journal of Psychoanalysis, 45*(2–3), 332–337.
Rosenfeld, H. (1971). A clinical approach to the psychoanalytic theory of the life and death instincts: An investigation into the aggressive aspects of narcissism. *The International Journal of Psychoanalysis, 52*, 169–178.
Rosenfeld, H. (1987). Afterthought: changing theories and changing techniques in psychoanalysis. In H. Rosenfeld (Ed.), *Impasse and interpretation* (pp. 273–288). Routledge.
Rothstein, A. (1999). *The narcissistic pursuit of perfection* (2nd rev. ed.). International Universities Press. (Original work published 1984)
Russ, E., Shedler, J., Bradley, R., & Westen, D. (2008). Refining the construct of narcissistic personality disorder: Diagnostic criteria and subtypes. *The American Journal of Psychiatry, 165*(11), 1473–1481. https://doi.org/10.1176/appi.ajp.2008.07030376

Sharp, C., Wright, A. G. C., Fowler, J. C., Frueh, B. C., Allen, J. G., Oldham, J., & Clark, L. A. (2015). The structure of personality pathology: Both general ('g') and specific ('s') factors? *Journal of Abnormal Psychology, 124*(2), 387–398. https://doi.org/10.1037/abn0000033

Smith, M. B., & Webster, B. D. (2018). Narcissus the innovator? The relationship between grandiose narcissism, innovation, and adaptability. *Personality and Individual Differences, 121*, 67–73. https://doi.org/10.1016/j.paid.2017.09.018

Symington, N. (1993). *Narcissism: A new theory*. Karnac Books.

Volkan, V. D. (1979). The "glass bubble" of the narcissistic patient. In J. LeBoit & A. Capponi (Eds.), *Advances in psychotherapy of the borderline patient* (pp. 405–431). Jason Aronson.

4 The theorists and their theories viewed through the lens of narcissism

"Psychiatric research, Freud noted, has no intention of denigrating the great and of 'dragging the sublime into the dust.' But Leonardo, 'already admired by his contemporaries as one of the greatest men of the Italian Renaissance,' is human like everyone else, and 'there is no one so great that it would be a disgrace for him to be subject to the laws that govern normal and pathological activity with equal severity.'"

(Gay, 1998, p. 283, citing Freud's 1916/2010 paper on Leonardo da Vinci)

Introduction

The narcissistic personality traits of Freud, Winnicott, and Kohut, as shaped by their formative life events and cultural and historical background, are discussed in this chapter based on the extensive psychobiographical literature on these three pioneers of psychoanalysis as well as on their own writings and correspondence. It is shown how their narcissistic personality traits colored their views and perceptions and limited the universality of their personality theories. The focus on the narcissistic personality traits of Freud, Winnicott, and Kohut may seem reductive considering the complex and unique personality, innovative thinking, and original contribution of each of these founding fathers of psychoanalysis. Yet given the crucial impact of their narcissistic position on psychoanalytic theory in its early days and its far-reaching implications, evident even in contemporary theory and clinical practice, I believe that the issue deserves serious consideration. Delving in depth, this chapter shows how the three core features of the narcissistic personality, namely, grandiosity, schizoidism, and the difficulty of acknowledging the otherness and separateness of the other, which serve as a self-protective shield against negative feelings, emotional vulnerability, and the ultimate collapse into an experience of the self as flawed and inferior, were manifested in the personalities of Freud, Winnicott, and Kohut and subsequently reflected in their theories.

Grandiosity is characterized by a sense of superiority and self-perfection. Also typical of the narcissistic grandiose position is a sense of uniqueness and entitlement. As shown, all these as well as identification with greater-than-life

DOI: 10.4324/9781003538295-4

figures, which is another characteristic of the grandiose personality, were displayed by Freud, Winnicott, and Kohut. Their grandiosity was reflected in their theories, inter alia, in the biased, self-enhancing criteria of mental health they proposed and in the key concepts they suggested that reinforced their sense of superiority. Yet, as discussed at length in my article on the split narcissist (Afek, 2018), the narcissist swings between defensive grandiosity, on the one end, and devastating feelings of vulnerability, imperfection, and inferiority, on the other extreme end of the narcissistic experience. As further shown, the dissociated self-experience of vulnerability, imperfection, and inferiority was also typical of the theorists under discussion and likewise points to their narcissistically defensive personality structure. In this context, the discussion focuses on the primary impact of their defensive grandiosity as it shaped their theories.

Schizoidism involves an illusory feeling of self-sufficiency and denial of the need for the other. As noted in Chapter 3, narcissistic schizoidism is not necessarily reflected in an overt behavior pattern of seclusion, but rather in denial of the emotional dependence on the other and avoidance of close intimate relationships. Indeed, the narcissist may be surrounded by people. However, his interpersonal relationships are superficial and merely functional. The narcissistic schizoidism of Freud, Winnicott, and Kohut is demonstrated based on their manifested preoccupation with their inner world, personal goals, and self-realization rather than with their interpersonal relationships. As shown, it was reflected in their theories in their excessive focus on the self and the fulfillment of its needs and in their associated failure to place due emphasis on the fundamental centrality of close emotional relationships in the human psyche.

The difficulty of acknowledging the otherness and separateness of the other is revealed in the failure to see the other as a separate subject with his own center of consciousness, views, perceptions, needs, and preferences as well as in the expectation that the other would adapt himself to the self and serve the self. It was clearly manifested in the difficulty of Freud, Winnicott, and Kohut recognizing the contribution of others to psychoanalysis, in general, and to their own theories, in particular, and further reflected in the elusive presence of the separate other in their theories.

Sigmund Freud – The bourgeois rebel

Sigmund (originally named Sigismund Schlomo) Freud was born in the small Moravian town of Freiberg in the Austrian Empire (now the Czech Republic) in 1856 to Jewish parents. He was the first son of his beautiful mother, who was 20 years younger than his father. It was the second (or even third) marriage of his father, who had two sons by his first marriage, one of them married with children. Throughout Sigmund's childhood, the family struggled financially as the father, who was a small trader, could not make ends meet notwithstanding his efforts. When Sigmund was about a year and a half old, his baby brother,

Julius, died in infancy, just seven months after birth. It may be assumed that his mother, overcome by grief over Julius and trying to cope with another loss upon the death of her brother around that time, was emotionally absent from Sigmund's life. When Freud was about two and a half years old, he was abruptly separated from another mother figure with the sudden disappearance of his nanny, who was indicted on theft charges and sentenced to prison time. No doubt, the loss, whether emotional or actual, of significant attachment figures so early in his life was a formative childhood experience that left an enduring mark on his personality. At the age of four years, Freud moved with his family to Vienna, where he spent most of his life, until he escaped the Nazi regime, fleeing to London in 1938, a year before his death.

Being an exceptionally gifted boy, Sigmund was idolized by his family. As a child prodigy, he enjoyed his mother's preferential attitude and was favored over his five younger sisters and little brother, Alexander, who were born one after the other. His grades at school were impressive, and as he himself proudly recounted (as cited by Gay, 1998, p. 19), "I was first in my class for seven years, held a privileged position, was scarcely ever examined." He was the only child who had a room of his own in the small house the family lived in. His sisters had to take care not to disturb him when he was studying, and the piano on which his sister Anna used to practice was promptly taken out so as not to bother him. He saw himself as an authoritative parental figure with respect to his sisters, and they had to obey him, for instance, when he decided that they should not read the supposedly provocative works of Balzac and Dumas.

Freud's mother was a dominant and domineering woman, while his father was mild-tempered and thus perceived as weak in the eyes of young Sigmund. The following episode, as related by Gay (1998), is illustrative of Freud's feelings about his father. During one of their walks together, Freud's father told his son of an encounter he had as a young fellow, when strolling down the street, an anti-Semitic Christian passing by knocked off his new fur cap into the mud, shouting, "Jew, off the sidewalk!" The father's meek reaction – "I stepped into the road and picked up my cap." – clearly disappointed the then teenaged Sigmund, and as he recalled, his father's submissiveness "did not seem heroic to me" (p. 9). Freud's identification through life with valiant heroes and gallant warriors is thus not surprising. One of the great historical figures Freud identified with was Hannibal, the Semitic Carthaginian general and statesman known for his lifelong struggle against the mighty Roman Republic. As Gay further noted, Freud "elevated him [Hannibal] into a symbol of 'the contrast between the tenacity of Jewry and the organization of the Catholic Church'" (pp. 9–10).

After graduating from high school, Freud decided to study medicine, aspiring to engage in research. He spent some time in a zoological research station, dissecting eels and exploring their reproductive organs; dedicated several years to brain research; and published various research papers on the nervous system and neuropathology, including studies on aphasia and cerebral palsy in children. Eventually, due to economic constraints, Freud turned to private clinical practice and opened a clinic for patients with nervous disorders. Basically, Freud was research oriented and less of a clinician – an orientation that was reflected in his essentially investigative therapeutic approach, which was aimed at uncovering underlying truths and corroborating his theory of the human psyche, at times, at the expense of empathy for the suffering of his patients.

At the age of 30, Freud married Martha, following four long years of courtship, in the course of which Freud sought to establish himself professionally and financially before starting a family. It was then that the romantic side of his personality was revealed. However, while ardently courting his fiancée, "my princess," as he called her when they were still engaged, his interest in her waned after their wedding. Once they got married, Martha was assigned the role of a mere helpmate. As a glamourless although efficient housewife, her main job was to take care of her genius husband and spare him the tedious task of dealing with everyday affairs. Freud had no doubt that he was the master of the house, the figure in authority with the right of decision regarding their life together. Thus, for instance, he forbade Martha to light the Shabbat candles or celebrate the Jewish holidays, which was not easy for her as she came from an Orthodox home. Yet she humbly accepted his requests. Her docile and compliant attitude may explain how they managed to get along together without ever coming into conflict (at least according to her). They had six children, born in succession, Mathilde, Jean-Martin, Oliver, Ernst, Sophie, and Anna, named by Freud himself after his admired role models or significant figures in his life. The Freud family lived in a nice and comfortable house, simply and conservatively furnished, and led a strictly disciplined bourgeois life. Martha firmly managed the house, attending to its routine maintenance and preparing gourmet meals. Her sister Minna, who moved in with the Freuds after the death of her fiancé, helped Martha with the household chores. Minna maintained a close friendly relationship with Freud, and there were rumors of a love affair between the two, so far, unsubstantiated. Freud was busy conducting research and working with his patients, usually following a fixed routine, going to sleep around 1 a.m., getting up at 7 a.m., seeing his patients or writing down his ideas until 1 p.m., when the family met for lunch, walking through the streets of Vienna after lunch, and seeing more patients until the evening hours. Freud made it a point to visit his mother, who was living nearby, every Saturday (his father passed away years before her). Saturday afternoons he gave lectures at the University of Vienna, and in the evening he used to meet with friends for a Tarock card game.

Freud was attached to his children, cared for them and loved them in his matter-of-fact, unemotional way. His children were disciplined and acquiescent and never challenged his authority. He was attentive to their concerns, offered his advice, and used to take them on vacations, which, of course, were carefully planned in advance. Occasionally, he shared his worries about them and, at times, his admiration of their brilliance in his extensive correspondence with colleagues and friends. "Annarel is developing charmingly; she is of Martin's type, physically and mentally," he wrote, delighted, in one of his letters to his friend Wilhelm Fliess (as cited by Gay, 1998, p. 98).

Freud had to struggle for financial survival most of his life to ensure a relatively stable and comfortable life for himself and his family. The threat of falling into poverty was always present, looming over, haunting him since his childhood. And it was not only the memory of his childhood under the shadow of penury that plagued him. Raising a family of six children was not an easy task, all the more so given the long hours of reading, writing, holding meetings, engaging in intellectual debates with colleagues, and fine-tuning his theory, entailed by his monumental psychoanalytic project.

When Freud was 40, his father passed away. The loss affected him profoundly, and as he wrote to Fliess in response to his friend's letter of condolences, "I now have a quite uprooted feeling" (Gay, 1998, p. 86). Reflecting on his father's death, Freud (1913) noted in the preface to the second edition of *The Interpretation of Dreams* that it was "the most significant event, the deepest loss, in the life of a man" (p. viii). Freud's intense reaction to the loss was remarkable and unexpected, especially considering his ambivalent feelings about his father. It seems that the death of his father motivated him to undergo self-analysis and write this groundbreaking work, which, as he noted in that context, had a "subjective meaning," perceived only after its completion. "It proved to be for me a part of my self-analysis, a reaction to the death of my father" (p. viii). While Freud was overwhelmed by his father's death, he reacted to the death of his mother many years later, when she was 95, in an emotionally detached manner. This could be attributed to her advanced age and his more mature stage in life, but also to his deep-seated negative feelings about her, which could be traced back to the emotional abandonment that he experienced in early childhood. As noted in Chapter 2, seeking to shield himself against recurrent abandonment, Freud resorted to denial of his negative feelings and idealization of the relationship between mother and son as the most perfect of all human relationships.

Along the way, as Freud was formulating his psychoanalytic theory, he adopted a series of mentors and associates, drawing on their clinical work in developing his theory. One of these was Josef Breuer, who was older than Freud by 14 years and, in a sense, offered his patronage to the ambitious and passionate young man. As it turned out, Breuer was to play a pivotal role in the birth of psychoanalysis. The partnership between the two yielded their seminal collaborative work *Studies on Hysteria* (Breuer & Freud, 1895/1995), which was largely based on Breuer's work with a patient known as Anna O. (Bertha Pappenheim), a case that inspired Freud's approach to psychoanalytic clinical practice. The young woman, who was 21 years old when first admitted to treatment, complained about various symptoms (persistent cough, language disorders, hallucinations, partial paralyses, and more), and Breuer found that when she was encouraged to talk about her thoughts and emotions, her symptoms were mitigated or even disappeared. For instance, when for some time, she could not bring herself to drink water no matter how thirsty she was, the symptom disappeared once she recalled that she had seen her lady companion letting her dog drink water out of a glass. This "talking cure," as labeled by Breuer, or "chimney sweeping," as Anna O. called it, led Freud to conclude that recollection and verbalization of repressed memories acted cathartically to relieve mental suffering.

At the age of 46, Freud established a discussion group, the Psychological Wednesday Circle, known later on as the Vienna Psychoanalytic Society, with the aim of developing his psychoanalytic theory. Originally comprising a number of young Viennese physicians, the group composition changed over the years, when others interested in Freud's ideas joined it while former followers dropped out or were expelled. The group convened at Freud's apartment every Wednesday afternoon and after being served coffee and cookies, held heated discussions on issues related to psychoanalytic theory, shrouded in cigarette and cigar smoke. Future luminaries, such as Alfred Adler, Otto Rank, and Wilhelm Stekel as well as Max Graf, the father of "Little Hans" (the subject of one of Freud's famous case studies), who became himself a psychoanalyst, were among the participants. Freud, who was an authoritative and even authoritarian figure, expected the group members to indisputably accept the tenets of his theory, in particular, his thesis of infantile and childhood sexuality and the Oedipal complex as governing the human psyche. Any of them who dared challenge Freud's ideas was denounced as a "traitor" or a "paranoid," a label freely employed by Freud, and banished from the group. Sooner or later, Freud distanced himself from former disciples, adherents, and colleagues who were at odds with him over issues of theory or practice. Even highly significant figures in his life like Josef Breuer, Freud's caring mentor early in his career and partner and associate in the study of hysteria; Carl Jung, whom Freud had seen as his successor; and Fliess, whom Freud had considered his closest friend, were cut off from his life when they raised doubts about his key concepts and ideas.

While Freud enjoyed international recognition and acclaim and witnessed the growing success of the psychoanalytic project, the last two decades of his life were fraught with hardship and pain. When he approached the age of 60, World War I broke out. During the four-year-long war, Freud and his family, like other Viennese residents, went hungry, suffering from a shortage of staple foods and other basic commodities. Potatoes, coats, and shoes were in scarce supply, and heating materials were nowhere to be found. Freud was sitting in his room shivering in the cold, looking in frustration for a usable fountain pen, trying to put his thoughts to paper, which was also scarce. His three sons served on the frontline and, naturally, he was anxious for their safety as well as for the safety of his sons-in-law and nephews. His son Martin was wounded in battle, taken captive by the Italians, and held in captivity for several months. One of his nephews, the son of his sister Rosa, was killed in the war (Rosa suffered another loss when her daughter committed suicide after becoming pregnant out of wedlock). In 1920, not long after the end of the war, Freud lost his beloved daughter Sophie, who died of pneumonia at the age of 27, and three years later, he lost his cherished grandson, Sophie's son, Heinele, who died of tuberculosis. The death of his dearly loved grandson was a terrible shock to Freud. "I am taking this loss so badly, I believe that I have never experienced anything harder," he wrote. "Fundamentally everything has lost its value" (Gay, 1998, p. 443). Around that time, Freud was diagnosed with cancer of the palate and suffered severe pain. A series of surgeries provided temporary relief but failed to substantially improve his condition, causing him even more severe pain, until, beaten by the disease, he passed away at the age of 83. The onset of World War II, when Freud was 80, did not make it any easier for him. The atmosphere on the streets of Vienna under Hitler was intimidating, rife with anti-Semitic persecution, attacks on Jewish institutions and Jews themselves, and unwarranted arrests, including that of Freud's daughter Anna, who was detained and interrogated in the cellars of the Gestapo. The times were so bad that Anna raised the option of suicide as a way out. However, Freud, who was not the type to give up hope and capitulate, ruled out the notion. It was only following the intervention of various personages, among them Princess Marie Bonaparte, who was a close friend of Freud, that Freud and his family received exit visas and emigrated to England.

Freud was a man of sharp contrasts – on the one hand, a staunch conservative striving for stability and seeking to maintain the existing order and, on the other hand, a bold trailblazer who managed to shake and transform Western culture. Freud believed in rationality, abhorred irrationality, and showed contempt for whatever could not be logically proven, including superstitions, illusions, religious dogmas, and so on. However, on occasion, he toyed with numerology, was troubled by the occult significance of certain numbers, experimented with telepathy together with Anna, and even wrote on the topic. And for all the gloom and seriousness that characterized him, his witty humor was occasionally revealed. Thus, when leaving Vienna in panic, escaping Nazi terror, Freud was required to sign a document declaring that he was treated well by the Nazi regime and had no complaints against the authorities. Freud signed the statement, sarcastically adding in handwriting, "I can most highly recommend the Gestapo to everyone" (Gay, 1998, p. 657).

Freud's narcissistic personality traits

Sándor Ferenczi, who was briefly analyzed by Freud, noted with reference to his analysis that Freud diagnosed himself as a narcissist (Ferenczi & Dupont, 1988):

> My own analysis could not be pursued deeply enough because my analyst (by his own admission, of a narcissistic nature), with his strong determination to be healthy and his antipathy toward any weaknesses or abnormalities, could not follow me down into those depths, and introduced the "educational" stage too soon.
>
> (p. 119)

Freud's grandiosity

Already as a young man, Freud was convinced that he was destined for greatness. When he was not yet 30, he confidently assured Martha, then his fiancée, in one of the letters he sent her that some day he would be featured in a laudatory biography as a man of great stature. He therefore destroyed various documents from his past, lest they fall into undesirable hands. Early on in his career, while he was busy writing *The Interpretation of Dreams*, Freud wondered in a letter to his then close friend Fliess, "Do you really believe that some day, on this house, one will read on a marble tablet: 'Here revealed itself, on July 24, 1895, the secret of the dream to Dr. Sigm. Freud'?" (Gay, 1998, p. 79). When still a student, Freud entertained similar fantasies of recognition and fame, envisioning his statue placed one day next to those of revered ex-professors adorning the university campus. And before reaching the age of 40, at the beginning of his career, Freud likened himself to Robert Koch, the discoverer of the pathogen of tuberculosis, claiming credit for the "discovery" of the etiology of hysteria.

Throughout his life, even as a child, Freud identified with greater-than-life figures. Thus, he imagined himself as Oedipus, the mythological Greek king of Thebes, who overcame the Sphinx by solving her riddle, lifting the Sphinx's curse off the Thebans. Another one of his adored heroes was Hannibal, who pledged to never be a friend of Rome but at no time approached nor conquered its capital. Freud identified with the legendary Carthaginian general so intensely that held back by "phobic prohibition" (Gay, 1998, p. 137), he refrained for years from visiting the Eternal City. Moses, leader of the Israelites, was another figure of identification for Freud. Comparing himself to Moses, who coming down from Mount Sinai with the tablets of the testimony, found his people worshipping the golden calf, Freud saw himself as a modern-day visionary whose revolutionary psychoanalytic theory was not duly appreciated by the ignorant common masses. Eventually, Freud visited and revisited Rome, never failing to call on the *Moses of Michelangelo*, carefully observing the magnificent marble sculpture, measuring its various parts, and contemplating its significance. Freud finally concluded, contrary to the traditional interpretation and the biblical story itself, that the tense facial expression of Michelangelo's *Moses* did not reflect uncontrollable fury at the sight of his people dancing around the golden calf idol, just as he was about to shatter the tablets of the testimony, but rather restrained rage, pointing to impressive abilities of self-control and sublimation – virtues that Freud boasted of possessing. His identification with Moses is further illustrated in his well-known statement in a letter to Jung, who was his disciple at the time and whom Freud saw then as his spiritual heir. "If I am Moses, then you are Joshua and we will take possession of the promised land of psychiatry, which I shall only be able to glimpse from afar" (Ferris, 1997, p. 244). Other illustrious figures admired by Freud were Copernicus, who demonstrated that the Sun rather than Earth was at the center of the universe, and Darwin, who suggested that all species, animals and humans alike, shared a common ancestry, thereby deflating human self-centeredness and sense of superiority. Freud (1920) prided himself on dealing an even bitter blow – the mightiest, as he conceitedly believed – to human narcissism and pretentious claim to rationality, proposing that the brutish animalistic drives of humans were central to and actually governed the human psyche.

Freud's grandiosity was also reflected in his condescending view of others. As a young man, he wrote in a letter to his fiancée that the "psychology of the common man is rather different from ours" (Gay, 1998, p. 551). He saw his fellow humans, with a few exceptions, as lazy, irrational, uncouth riffraff. "I . . . experience a strong inclination to surrender to my affects, and feel strengthened in my whole unscientific position that when all is said, on the average, all things considered, human beings are miserable rabble," Freud wrote to Arnold Zweig (Gay, 1998, p. 609). Freud looked down on the lower classes, considered Eastern European Jews inferior, and disparaged the Americans as foolish, uneducated materialists who worshipped the dollar. Freud's chauvinistic view of women is well known. Thus, for instance, he saw women as morally inferior to men, believed that women should devote their time and energy to housekeeping and to raising and educating their children rather than go out to work, and regarded as absurd the idea of women's emancipation. "It seems a completely unrealistic notion to send women into the struggle for existence in the same way as men. Am I to think of my delicate sweet girl a competitor?" he wrote to Martha while still engaged to her (Masson, 1988/2012, p. 296). At the same time, Freud cultivated close relationships with a number of brilliant women, among them Lou Andreas-Salomé and Princess Marie Bonaparte, but his attitude toward them was the exception that proves the rule. Nonconformist and groundbreaking as Freud was, he subscribed to the contemporary deprecative view of women, which was compatible with his narcissistic need to associate himself with the superior class of men. His attitude toward his patients was similarly derogatory and even exploitative – an attitude typical of the narcissistic personality. As noted by Ferenczi (Ferenczi & Dupont, 1988), citing Freud under the heading "Doctor hating patients," Freud saw the latter as "rabble . . . only any good for making money out of, and for studying" (p. 118). While denigrating entire population groups and disdainfully referring to the masses as the "miserable rabble," who lacked sublimation, Freud saw himself as a refined, enlightened man who managed to rise above the primitive instinctual impulses that control the common folk – a self-concept that enhanced his sense of superiority.

Likewise characteristic of Freud's grandiosity was his failure to comply with his own recommendation to the analyst to maintain the boundaries vis-à-vis the analysand. He psychoanalyzed the lover of Ferenczi, the spouse of his biographer Ernest Jones, and, most notoriously, his own daughter Anna and her sexual phantasies. His failure to maintain the boundaries between therapist and patient reflects his narcissistic sense of entitlement, and hence his haughty disregard of the norms and standards required of ordinary people but not binding, as he believed, the exceptional, ingenious, privileged few.

Freud saw himself as the elder of the tribe, the senior leader outlining the way for his colleagues in the Psychological Wednesday Circle, who were expected to devoutly follow his doctrine. Indeed, Freud shaped the group along the lines of a religious cult and presented rings to those he deemed worthy of participating in his exclusive circle of the privileged, as a token of their allegiance. It is worth noting in this context that Stekel saw Freud as a noble figure, the like of Jesus, and himself as Freud's apostle (Strozier, 2001). In those early days, the Wednesday Circle offered Freud the backing he needed, sustaining his grandiose sense of superiority.

Freud's vulnerable, inferior, dissociated sense of self

Jones, who knew Freud for years and became his official biographer, noted (as cited by Gay, 1998, p. 156) that Freud's "profound self-confidence had been masked by strange feelings of inferiority, even in the intellectual sphere." As further noted by Gay, based on Jones, Freud sought to overcome these feelings "by elevating his mentors to an unassailable position, which then permitted him to remain dependent upon them" (p. 156). Freud's sense of inferiority was evident in his relations with idealized colleagues and associates. Occasionally, he had to bolster his self-confidence with a dose of cocaine (which he often used to lift his spirits), for instance, when he was about to meet eminent French neurologist Jean-Martin Charcot, by whom Freud was "dazzled" (p. 46). His relationship with Fliess was similarly marked by self-effacement. Thus, in a letter to his friend, dated October 3, 1897, Freud humbly wrote, *I hope to be offered some more crumbs off your table*, and in another letter, dated August 6, 1899, Freud rhetorically asked, *Dear Wilhelm, Do you ever go wrong?* (Rolnik, 2019). Freud's insecurity was likewise reflected in his letters to his fiancée. While courting her, "he wondered whether he was really worthy of his Martha. She was, he told her over and over, his princess, but he often doubted that he was a prince" (Gay, 1998, p. 38). At the same time, he was possessive about her and jealous of any person emotionally close to her and, as noted by Gay, his efforts to monopolize her attested to his "wavering self-esteem" (p. 39).

Freud had a strange recurring dream of a humiliating childhood incident that occurred when he was about eight years old and "urinated in his parents' bedroom, in their presence." The memory of his father, exasperated over his act of disrespect, telling him "that he would never amount to anything" haunted Freud for years, and he recalled it as a "terrible blow to my ambition" (Gay, 1998, p. 21). Yet as further related by Gay, when the scene was persistently replayed in Freud's dreams, he countered by enumerating "his successes, as though to show his father, triumphantly, that he had amounted to something after all" (p. 21). I believe that recurring dreams have a special significance as they revolve around unresolved, deep-seated issues that are processed over and over again in the dream. Freud was evidently deeply uncertain about his self-worth and thus had to repeatedly remind himself of his achievements. His profound insecurity is reflected in another dream that evoked a minor and apparently insignificant episode, where Freud was strolling along the shoreline during a visit to his half brother Emmanuel, who was living in England. Meeting a little girl on the way who asked him something about a starfish, Freud replied in English, using the pronoun "he" instead of "it" to refer to the starfish. He was so deeply embarrassed by the slight grammatical mistake that he kept dreaming about it for years. Any failure, small as it might have been, presented a threat to his self-worth or could even lead to a total collapse of his self-esteem, so that his grandiose self-experience had to be restored over and over again.

Freud's insecurity was also reflected in his feeling that the people he met did not like him and tended to underestimate him, as he wrote in a letter to Martha dated January 17, 1886 (Rolnik, 2019). It may be assumed that Freud attributed to others his lowly self-perception of inferiority and imperfection. Aron and Starr (2013) ascribed Freud's feelings of inferiority to the rampant anti-Semitism of his era, which deprecated Jewish men as flawed and castrated, irrational, and immoral. Freud's ambivalence about his Jewishness, apparently indicative of unconscious self-hate, could thus be traced back to the prevalent anti-Semitic ideology of the time (Boyarin et al., 2003). While Freud did not deny his Jewishness, his ambivalence regarding his Jewish identity was manifested in various ways. Thus, Freud tended to draw on ancient Greek mythology rather than on the Hebrew Bible. He was hostile toward Eastern European Jews, who were seen by him as inferior (although he himself was born to Jewish parents of Eastern European origin). He ignored the Jewish background of his patients, taking no account of the anti-Semitic society they lived in and its relevance to their situation. When it came to naming his children, as Aron and Starr (2013) noted, "Freud named all his sons after famous non-Jews, and all his daughters after Jewish women," which indicated "his unconscious ambivalence about his Jewishness" (p. 192). Also, Freud asserted, strangely enough, that Moses – one of his figures of identification – was actually an Egyptian (murdered by the Israelites, who crowned another Hebrew Canaanite Moses in his place). And he was firmly against celebrating the Jewish holidays while allowing the celebration of Christmas and Easter in the family circle.

Freud's split personality

The dreams of Freud, extensively discussed by him in *The Interpretation of Dreams* (Freud, 1913), open a window into his inner world and provide ample material on his split personality. His dissociated self-states, fluctuating between a grandiose self-experience, on the one hand, and an experience of the self as flawed and inferior, on the other hand, are clearly reflected in the Hercules dream, as I label it. In his dream, Freud saw a bench covered with little heaps of excrement. He urinated on the bench and the stream of urine rinsed it clean. The trigger for the dream was a lecture that Freud gave that evening, with which he was displeased, feeling that it was a failure. He was dissatisfied with himself, tired and dispirited. The unconscious phantasies evoked in his dream by association led him, inter alia, to King Augeas's stables, which, as the Greco-Roman myth goes, were cleansed by Hercules, who, using his legendary strength, diverted the rivers Alpheios and Pineios through the stables. Analyzing his dream, Freud identified himself as the mythological hero Hercules, while other associations were evoked suggestive of his greatness and the honor accorded him by his appreciative patients. Along with the illusions of megalomania, Freud identified in his dream delusions of inferiority. The heaps of excrement apparently symbolized his deep-rooted experience of the self as inferior, while Hercules and other heroic figures that populated his dream, among them Gulliver, signified his grandiose, omnipotent sense of self. The dream is thus indicative of Freud's dissociated sense of self, which at the slightest failure, whether real or imagined (in this case, a lecture perceived by Freud as unsuccessful), was liable to collapse into a self-experience of vulnerability, imperfection, and inferiority. The narcissistic compensatory defense mechanism of self-aggrandizement was thus employed by Freud in the face of the looming collapse of his precarious self-esteem.

The following passage by Freud (1914/1955), describing his feelings in front of Michelangelo's sculpture of Moses in the church of San Pietro in Vincoli in Rome, provides further illustration of his dissociated sense of self:

> Sometimes I have crept cautiously out of the half-gloom of the interior as though I myself belonged to the mob upon whom his eye is turned – the mob which can hold fast no conviction, which has neither faith nor patience, and which rejoices when it has regained its illusory idols.
>
> (p. 213)

As Freud himself admitted, he occasionally experienced himself as one of the inferior, ignorant riffraff, the unfaithful mob that traded the Law of God for a golden idol, rejecting the Ten Commandments brought down from Mount Sinai by "Moses, the Law-giver of the Jews" (p. 213) – the Moses whom Freud adored and with whom he identified.

Freud's split self-perception was also reflected in his polarized evaluation of his own writings. Thus, for instance, in a letter to Ferenczi, dated December 16, 1910, written by Freud upon completion of his paper on the case of Schreber, Freud wondered whether his analysis of the German judge's account of his nervous illness would be met with stinging ridicule or rather win him universal acclaim, or perhaps draw both scorn and applause (Rolnik, 2019). It appears that Freud could not imagine a moderate reaction to his work, projecting onto others his fragmented self-perception as either a glorified figure or an inferior, ignoble character, one of the mob. The sharp fluctuations between the two extreme poles of his sense of self were variously discussed in the literature. Rudnytsky (1991) referred to Freud's "oscillation between 'delusions of inferiority' and 'megalomania' in his own self-esteem"

(p. 135). Gay (1998) cited Freud's own description of himself as "in turn proud and blissful, embarrassed and miserable" and further noted that Freud was given to "the most wildly oscillating fantasies of fame and failure" (p. 75). An episode cited by Aron and Starr (2013) from Freud's 1919 *The "Uncanny"* is similarly indicative of his dissociated sense of self. As related by Freud, while riding a train, sitting alone in his wagon-lit compartment, he thought that his reflection in the mirror was an intruder, but soon realized to his dismay that it was his own reflection in the looking-glass, which he "thoroughly disliked." By experiencing his own image as alien, the authors noted, Freud turned away from the "disliked, uncanny aspects of himself" (p. 298), projecting his inferior self onto others.

The impact of Freud's grandiosity on his theory

The main axis around which Freud's psychoanalytic theory revolves is the Oedipal complex, unfolding in early childhood, between the ages of three and five, specifically during the development of a young boy. Centered on the son's incestuous desire for the mother and rivalry with and death wish against the father, who is perceived by the son as a threatening figure triggering castration anxiety, the Freudian Oedipal drama wraps up with the son's renunciation of his desire for his mother and internalization of his father's values. The Oedipal complex, depicted by Freud as regulating male psychology, reflects his narcissistic need to see himself as a phallic male, a fierce heroic warrior, who, like Oedipus, is possessed by sexual desire and capable of killing his father. The emphasis on the "phallic male" is intentional and significant. Freud could not conceive of himself as a vulnerable little child who depends on maternal breastfeeding (Ferenczi & Dupont, 1988; Sprengnether, 2003), nor could he see himself as a hapless baby abandoned to his death by his parents like the mythological Oedipus, who when just born, was left to die on a mountainside. The real foe visualized by Freud was the father figure rather than another child of equal standing. Accordingly, it was the conflict between the little child (even if merely imagined) and the paternal male figure of authority rather than sibling rivalries that Freud saw as critical in psychological development. Freud felt compelled to deny not only the child in him but also other aspects of his personality that reflected vulnerability, helplessness, and inferiority, regarded by him as feminine (Sprengnether, 2003). Illustrative of Freud's emphasis on his masculinity, denial of his vulnerability and inferiority, and rejection of any association of himself with allegedly feminine or maternal traits is his comment, reported by one of his patients, American poet Hilda Doolittle (as cited by Aron & Starr, 2013, p. 298), "I do not like to be the mother in the transference – it always surprises and shocks me a little. I feel so very masculine." His view of women as inferior and flawed, and hence his portrayal of the young girl in the Oedipal drama as lacking and therefore envious of the male penis and as morally underdeveloped enabled him to sustain his self-image as a privileged member of the superior gender of males.

Freud clung to rationality and saw it as the only acceptable, practical, mature way of negotiating life challenges. Thus, as Gay (1998) noted, "This practical cast of mind inevitably shaped Freud's rather distant and quizzical relationship to music" (p. 173), which, as Freud felt, stirred vague, irrational, and uncontrollable emotions. Rationality and the ability to sublimate instinctual impulses were seen by Freud as indicative of a high level of personal development. As a self-proclaimed civilized man of reason possessing self-control and sublimation abilities, Freud considered himself a paragon of mental health. Accordingly, Freud defined mental health criteria and set therapeutic goals. Thus, for instance, his own depressive tendencies and habitual gloomy mood were perceived by him as a normal phenomenon that had to be put up with. True to his elitist approach, Freud "created a psychotherapy to match," adapted to highly intelligent and civilized patients, that is, individuals endowed with superior qualities, just like him, who could benefit from his exclusive, superb psychoanalysis, as otherwise, "If the physician has to deal with a worthless character, he soon loses the interest which makes it possible for him to enter profoundly into the patient's mental life" (Ferris, 1997, p. 198).

Freud's schizoidism

Freud identified to a large extent with the "primal father of the horde" (Freud, 1921, p. 124), the earliest indisputable leader of mankind, who was characterized by self-centeredness, absolute independence, and a lack of sympathy for others. As described in Freud's own words, "the leader himself need love no one else, he may be of a masterful nature, absolutely narcissistic, self-confident and independent" (pp. 123–124). And that was the way Freud chose to see himself, as emotionally self-sufficient, free of any dependence, and assured of himself. Indeed, as suggested by Edmundson (2007), Freud had "a mild misanthropy" that accounted, in part, for his dog obsession (p. 91). In this context, Edmundson cited Hilda Doolittle as complaining that when analyzed by Freud, he seemed to be more interested in his dog than in her story. Likewise, Ferenczi noted that Freud "no longer loves his patients" and that he became interested solely in himself and in his scientific work (Ferenczi & Dupont, 1988, p. xxiv). It seems that Freud would have agreed with his portrayal by Ferenczi as a "scientific investigator" (p. xxiv) with a primarily intellectual interest in his psychoanalytic project. Actual interpersonal relationships were of less interest to him, and the same is true for his work as a therapist, which he carried on due to financial constraints while using his patients as objects for psychological research. In a letter from September 1875, Freud confessed to Eduard Silberstein, his most intimate friend at the time, "Last year, asked what my greatest wish might be, I would have answered: a laboratory and free time, or a ship on the ocean with all the instruments the researcher needs" (Gay, 1998, p. 24). A glorious fantasy of schizoid isolation far out at sea, far away from human company! In fact, the schizoid fantasy was far removed from Freud's real life as he was always surrounded by people. However, his relation to others was essentially functional and emotionally distant, and he was not really concerned with the people around him, with their lives, or with their feelings. What interested him most of all were his own projects. His detached attitude toward others was reflected in his position on the therapist-patient relationship. Sharing with Martha his thoughts on "the physician's need to keep his emotional distance from all patients," he wrote her in one of his letters, when still at the beginning of his career,

> I could well imagine how painful it was for you to hear how I sit by a sickbed in order to observe, how I treat human suffering as an object. But my girl, it can't be done any other way and must look different to me than to others.
>
> (Gay, 1998, p. 37)

His position did not change over the years and was reaffirmed later on in his career, inter alia, in a postscript written in 1927 to *The Question of Lay Analysis* (Freud, 1926):

> I have no knowledge of having had any craving in my early childhood to help suffering humanity. . . . I scarcely think, however, that my lack of a genuine medical temperament has done much damage to my patients. For it is not greatly to the advantage of patients if their doctor's therapeutic interest has too marked an emotional emphasis. They are best helped if he carries out his task coolly and keeping as closely as possible to the rules.
>
> (pp. 253–254)

Throughout his life, Freud saw his patients as a source of research data and as objects for his studies. He was less concerned with their suffering or with them as real human beings who deserved empathy. Ferenczi cited Freud as noting on more than one occasion that "neurotics are a rabble, good only to support us financially and to allow us to learn from their cases" (Ferenczi & Dupont, 1988, p. 186). Freud sought to rationalize his emotionally distant attitude as a therapist, claiming, as noted, that it was beneficial to his patients. He believed that the psychoanalyst should adopt a dispassionate approach devoid of any personal or emotional involvement. Yet it seems that his position in the matter had to do with his own difficulty with intimacy in the therapeutic setting. As Freud himself admitted, he "did not like to be looked at all day" by his patients and preferred to sit "out of sight" behind the analytic couch (Aron, 1996, p. 141).

Freud's focus on his own personal issues and affairs and on his psychoanalytic research rather than on the significance of his interpersonal relationships is clearly reflected in his interpretation of his dreams. For the most part, his interpretations centered on wishes related to his professional standing, self-identity, masculine image, achievements, Oedipal conflicts, and so on, while overlooking pre-Oedipal issues such as emotional dependence, abandonment anxiety, rejection anxiety, and emotional intimacy. Thus, the two main dreams discussed by Freud (1913) in *The Interpretation of Dreams*, the dream of Irma's injection and the dream of the botanical monograph, were interpreted by Freud as related to his need for achievement, to his career aspirations, and to his concerns about his professional status. At the same time, alternative interpretations suggest that interpersonal relationships and the need for emotional intimacy with the other are, in fact, the underlying themes of Freud's dreams.

In the dream of Irma's injection, Freud meets Irma, a former patient, in a party and learns from her that she still suffers from various symptoms, which could of course mean that he failed to cure her. As the dream unfolds, Freud absolves himself of responsibility for Irma's condition, laying the blame on others, specifically a colleague who gave her a dubious injection using an unsterile syringe. Analyzing his dream, Freud concluded that the dream reflected his wish to exonerate himself and restore his professional self-esteem – clearly, an untypical Freudian interpretation. Sprengnether (2003) offered a completely different interpretation, arguing that Freud's analysis of the dream "reveals his preoccupation with issues of mastery and competence – both 'masculine' or phallic concerns" while "aspects of the dream that associate him with Irma" – notably, the bleeding they both suffered following nasal surgery performed by Fliess – pointed to the passive, submissive, vulnerable aspects of Freud's personality, which he regarded as feminine and thus chose to deny (p. 259). As Sprengnether further noted, "Irma's mouth, both the sign of her 'femininity' and the dream's imagistic center, offers a point of departure for an oral (as opposed to phallic) interpretation" (p. 260).

The dream of the botanical monograph was described by Freud (1913) in a few words, as follows:

> I have written a monograph on a certain plant. The book lies before me. I am just turning over a folded coloured plate. A dried specimen of the plant is bound up with every copy, as though from a herbarium.
>
> (p. 143)

The trigger for the dream was a monograph on the genus *Cyclamen* that Freud saw that day in the showcase of a bookstore. The stream of associations generated by that episode led Freud to analyze the dream as primarily dealing with his failure to publish in time a groundbreaking research paper written by him on the anesthetic properties of the coca plant and his subsequent loss of the recognition and acclaim he hoped for, eventually won by a colleague who had published the discovery before Freud managed to have his monograph issued. However, it seems to me, reflecting on the dream and the associations presented by Freud, that the dream is actually indicative of Freud's marital relationship with Martha and the strains on their relationship. The flowers appearing as a central image in the dream are a telltale sign. As noted by Freud, the cyclamen was the flower of choice of his wife, but he seldom remembered to bring her the flowers she liked, while she never failed to surprise him with his favorite artichoke flowers. Why was Freud so forgetful and failed to delight Martha once in a while with a bouquet of cyclamens? Was it his passive-aggressive attitude toward her, provoked by her emotionally frustrating position or by her failure to stimulate him intellectually? Or was it his preoccupation with himself that blinded him to her existence and needs? It is noteworthy that Dr. Koenigstein, who plays a key role in the dream, reproaches Freud for being too self-centered and too fond of his hobbies to be concerned with others. Or could it be that other women became an object of desire for Freud? Perhaps Mrs. Flora, whose name connotes a flower . . .

Both dreams are indicative of Freud's blindness to his own vulnerable self and to his deep-rooted need for an intimate interpersonal relationship. However, that's not the way Freud saw it. He interpreted both dreams as reflecting or enhancing his image as a phallic, achievement oriented male. His vulnerability and need for an emotionally close, supporting figure were hardly, if ever, referred to in his dream analyses. It should be noted, though, that in certain situations in life, Freud acknowledged his emotional need for the other and allowed himself the luxury of yearning for emotional intimacy, but this only when he was involved in a relationship that was out of reach and could not be realized or in a relationship that was otherwise perceived as idyllic. This was true for his relationship with Martha while they were still engaged, which, for several years, was conducted mainly by mail. Throughout that period, Freud was in a state of emotional excitement, longing to see his "princess," wondering whether he deserved her, fervently expressing his need for her and desire to meet her. But once they married and his remote, ideal object of desire became a real presence in his life, his passion cooled, and the romance faded away. Likewise, his relationship with Fliess, a once close friend whom Freud adored, looking up to him as an intimate confidant and a source of inspiration, came to an end when Fliess expressed independent views at variance with Freud and thus was no longer seen as the perfect associate Freud had believed him to be. The rift between the two was never healed.

The following observation by Freud (1960/1992) in a letter to Martha from August 29, 1883, early on in their acquaintance, could shed light on his need to keep his distance from others:

> Why don't we fall in love with a different person every month? Because at each separation a part of our heart would be torn away. Why don't we make a friend of everyone? Because the loss of him or any misfortune befalling him would affect us deeply. Thus, we strive more towards avoiding pain than seeking pleasure.
>
> (p. 50)

The impact of Freud's schizoidism on his theory

Freud's mechanistic view of the human psyche, drawing on 19th-century neurological research that described the mind as "a little machine fueled by electrical and chemical forces" and suggested "a physiological substratum for all mental events" (Gay, 1998, pp. 127–128), reflects his defensively reductionistic and materialistic view of human beings and their interpersonal relationships. Freud believed that relationships between individuals, children and adults alike, were egoistically driven by sexual and aggressive impulses rather than motivated by a deep-seated, inherent need for emotional intimacy, for sharing with other human beings, for empathy for others, and for generosity toward others. Manifestations of altruism were seen by him as a reaction formation against sadistic wishes, unacceptable sexual desire, or other denied negative or exploitative wishes or impulses (Strenger, 1989). The Oedipal complex around which the human psyche is organized, according to Freud, is all about envy, competitiveness, aggressiveness, sexuality, castration anxiety, or castration experience, while the quest for emotional intimacy, the need for love, feelings of longing, the enjoyment derived from interpersonal relationships, grief over loss, and the like are missing from the equation. The same is true for emotional attachment in the first years of infancy, which is not considered of primary significance in Freud's psychosexual development model. Rather, the infant's sexual and aggressive impulses and wishes and their gratification take center stage in Freud's drive theory. The parents are perceived by the infant as vague figures serving as objects for the projection of desires and wishes and the satisfaction of instincts rather than as unique human beings with whom unique and specific relationships are maintained. Schizoidism thus underlies the early stages of infantile development. The newborn is described as cut off from the external world, with the libido directed inward (primary narcissism). At the next stage, the infant's libido is directed toward the mother, who functions as a mere object for need fulfillment and has no distinct human presence. Her unique personality, feelings, wishes, and behavior patterns are seen as irrelevant, and the infant's relationship with her is a merely functional relationship between subject and object, devoid of emotional intimacy (similar, in a sense, to a need-based relationship between a man and a woman).

Freud's failure to take due account of the innate need for emotional attachment to a significant other is likewise reflected in his theorizing on loss and grief processes as well as in his clinical approach to the issue. Thus, as noted by Mitchell (1993), Freud ignored the loss-related intrapsychic dynamics of his patients, even when loss and mourning played a key role in their lives, focusing instead on their repressed sexuality. In *Mourning and Melancholia*, Freud (1917) discussed mourning as a normal mental process that came to an end with the withdrawal of the libido from the lost object of love (decathexis) and its displacement to another object, contrasting it with melancholia, which he saw as pathological. That is to say, emotional withdrawal from the lost object of love was seen by Freud as indicative of a normal and healthy mourning process – a view that plays down the significance of a unique, intimate relationship with a loved person, as if anyone is replaceable. It should be noted, though, that Freud subsequently presented a somewhat different view in *The Ego and the Id* (Freud, 1923), stating that the substitution of object cathexis by identification with the lost object of love, originally seen by him as indicative of pathological depression, namely, melancholia (Freud, 1917), was part of the conclusion of a normal mourning process. In other words, Freud acknowledged in his 1923 essay that a normal and healthy mourning process did not necessarily involve complete emotional detachment from the deceased. However, Freud never fully developed the idea in his theory, and to the extent that he referred to the internalization of the loved one's image in the mourner's ego, he did not enlarge on the mourner's continuing bond with the loved one as a separate object or on his grief over the loss. While Freud did not pursue the issue any further in his theoretical writings, his painful personal experience following the loss of his beloved daughter Sophie, when she was just 27, and the death of her son, his dearly loved grandson Heinele, three years afterward taught him otherwise. His agony following the loss of his grandson was unbearable, so much so that he lost his taste for life, and as he wrote to his friend Max Eitingon, he was "obsessed by impotent longing for the dear child" (Gay, 1998, p. 443). In a letter of condolence to his friend Ludwig Binswanger upon the death of Ludwig's eight-year-old son, dated April 11, 1929, Freud (1960/1992) explicitly stated that the gap left by the loss of a loved one could never be filled:

> Although we know that after such a loss the acute state of mourning will subside, we also know we shall remain inconsolable and will never find a substitute. No matter what may fill the gap, even if it be filled completely, it nevertheless remains something else. And actually this is how it should be. It is the only way of perpetuating that love which we do not want to relinquish.
>
> (p. 386)

Notwithstanding his own agonizing experience, it seems that Freud was not yet prepared to revise his theory or perhaps did not manage to accomplish such revision in the twilight of his life.

Freud developed a psychoanalytic clinical practice that encouraged emotional distance between therapist and patient. He saw the role of the therapist as that of an impartial, dispassionate scientist or surgeon and believed that the therapist should maintain a low-key presence, sitting out of sight behind the analytic couch, and thus avoid eye contact with the patient as far as possible. The Freudian clinical practice was focused on interpretations as the major agent of change. That is, the rational, intellectual, emotionally distant discourse rather than the close, emotional, experiential contact between therapist and patient was seen by Freud as most conducive to change.

Freud's difficulty acknowledging the otherness and separateness of the other

Freud expected those close to him, family members as well as friends and colleagues, to adapt themselves to his needs and wishes and, in effect, to serve as his extension. Thus, he expected his wife Martha to devote herself to the task of caring for him, her adored husband, and tending to all his needs so that he would be free to pursue his work and his psychoanalytic project. Furthermore, Freud required her to do as he wished in all areas of life and to completely identify with him, with his feelings and views. For instance, when still engaged to her, he expected her to emulate his hostile feelings toward her mother and not only distance herself from her mother but actually feel the same hostility toward her (Atwood & Stolorow, 1993, citing Jones, 1953). As previously noted, after their marriage, he banned Martha from keeping the Jewish traditions that were honored at her Orthodox parents' home and that she sought to preserve, such as Shabbat candle lighting, observing the Shabbat, and celebrating the Jewish holidays (e.g., Passover and the Jewish New Year), and as always, she submissively complied. Ignoring her and her wishes, Freud took the liberty of naming their children as he deemed fit without consulting her. Thus, Mathilde was named after the wife of his revered mentor Breuer, who warmly welcomed young and poor Freud as a guest at their home. Jean-Martin was named after Jean-Martin Charcot, an idolized inspirational figure who impressed and charmed Freud and, in particular, amazed him with his use of hypnotic suggestion to cure hysterical paralysis. Freud's other children were likewise named by him. Anna, the youngest of the clan, served as a caregiver for her father and, in fact, as his extension throughout his life, much like his wife Martha. Anna adored her father, took care of him as a compassionate nurse when he was diagnosed with pharyngeal cancer, and even fought his battles. Her "passionate feelings for her father" were clearly revealed in a dream she had when she was about 20, as related by her. "Recently I dreamt that you are a king and I a princess, that people want to separate us by means of political intrigues" (Gay, 1998, p. 461). She was his daughter, his analysand, his close assistant, and a theorist in her own right, who devoutly followed in his footsteps, consolidating his theory while never questioning his presumptions. Freud was well aware that his daughter's close association with him might stand in the way of her happiness. Indeed, Anna never married, and it seems that her absolute devotion to her father suited him. As noted by Edmundson (2007):

> Freud's behavior toward others can sometimes suggest that he nourished pronounced doubts about their actuality. . . . He was capable of comparing the prospect of Anna's moving away and abandoning him and Martha with his having to give up his cigars.
>
> (p. 129)

Similarly, Freud expected blind loyalty from his colleagues and associates. It seems that any disagreement with his ideas was a critical blow to his narcissistic ego that he could not sustain. Thus, Freud cut off his relationship with Breuer over theoretical differences of opinion, although, as noted, Freud owed him a lot. Breuer was a benevolent fatherly figure for Freud, supported him financially, opened his home to him, invited him for meals, let him take baths at his place, and even came to his defense when Freud was attacked by the Vienna Doctors Association, although Breuer doubted the validity of the ideas proposed by his young protégé. Most significantly, Breuer introduced Freud to the case of Anna O. and the "talking cure" (as contrasted with hypnotic techniques), and the rest is history. Breuer also introduced Freud to another key figure in his life, a young physician by the name of Wilhelm Fliess, who became a true friend and for several years was Freud's close confidant, lending an attentive ear to his theoretical reflections, his doubts, and his thoughts. In a sense, Fliess seems to have served as an idealized *selfobject* for Freud (to use the term coined by Kohut), this, until Fliess voiced opposing views, which provoked Freud's ire and led to his alienation from his once best friend. Freud's intolerance for divergent views was clearly manifested in his attitude toward his colleagues in the Psychological Wednesday Circle, who helped him in developing his psychoanalytic theory. Any member of the group who failed to fall into line and dared express independent opinions was summarily expelled as a "traitor" or a "paranoid." Fritz Wittles, a Viennese physician who joined the group several years later, aptly described it, noting that (as cited by Ferris, 1997), "Freud didn't want to be argued with. He wanted a kaleidoscope lined with mirrors that would multiply the images he introduced into it" (p. 188). Jung, who had been seen by Freud as the crown prince chosen to lead psychoanalysis as his successor, was cut off from his life when Jung raised doubts about Freud's drive theory, arguing, inter alia, that the libido should not be conceived as narrowly sexual, but rather regarded as a general mental energy involving various complex processes that underlie the human psyche. Jung further criticized Freud for treating his disciples in a way that produced "slavish sons" (Gay, 1998, p. 440). Adler, Stekel, Rank, and others who challenged Freud were likewise excluded from the group. Swiss psychiatrist Eugen Bleuler, who introduced the term and concept *schizophrenia*, chose to break with Freud and resign from the newly organized International Psychoanalytic Association, unwilling to put up with the "tightly controlled political machine" that Freud was building up. As he told Freud, "This 'who is not for us is against us'" approach could be "necessary for religious communities and useful for political parties . . . but for science I consider it harmful" (Gay, 1998, p. 221). In the same vein, Edmundson (2007) noted:

> Freud's treatment of his . . . disciples is a complex subject, but one could never mistake him for a humane and humorous, much less a loving, mentor. He sometimes appears to believe that his disciples were created for the exclusive purpose of developing his work and enhancing his reputation.
>
> (p. 129)

Freud was wary of discovering that others could outshine him with their theoretical contributions (Aron & Starr, 2013) and thus threaten his self-image of superiority and perfection. This was true not only for his colleagues and associates but even for figures that he did not know personally. Thus, "Freud once said that he had not read much of Nietzsche, virtually all of whose books he nonetheless owned, because he was afraid that in Nietzsche's work he would find too many of the truths of psychoanalysis anticipated" (Edmundson, 2007, p. 161). At the same time, those who adapted themselves to Freud's needs and wishes, adopted his ideas, and displayed unquestioning loyalty to him enjoyed a lasting and stable relationship with him. Ernest Jones, for one, was a loyal adherent of Freud. Jones helped Freud in organizing the International Psychoanalytic Association and never challenged his superior position. Indeed, Jones self-deprecatingly admitted that he had no pretension to originality or ingenuity (Ferris, 1997).

As noted, Freud's attitude toward his patients was similarly authoritarian, demanding, and inconsiderate of their personal perspectives and feelings. He expected them to indisputably accept his insights and interpretations and felt resentful when they disagreed with him or refused to play the game by his rules. He could not even consider the possibility that he was wrong and they were right. A case in point is that of Dora, who was referred to Freud's treatment by her father when she was 16. However, as related by Masson (1988/2012), rather than showing real interest in Dora's truth and accepting at face value her report of the sexual abuse that she had experienced when just 14, and then again later on, at the hands of Herr K., a family friend, Freud displayed an arrogant know-all attitude, with no empathy for her plight. Dora was all the more embittered by the feeling that instead of protecting her, her father had handed her over to Herr K. on a platter so that he would be able to lead an affair with Herr K.'s wife. Yet Freud "was actually concerned with proving his theory" (p. 11) regarding female sexuality and callously dismissed Dora's reported sexual abuse experience at the age of 14, when Herr K. forcibly embraced her and pressed a kiss on her lips, attributing her disgusted reaction to sexual excitement and repressed sexual desires. Thus, Freud "trivialized her deepest concern," stripping her experience of any significance (p. 14).

Freud's dismissive position in the therapeutic setting and failure to treat his patients as human beings and acknowledge their uniqueness and otherness were manifested in other spheres of life as well. Freud was antagonistic to unfamiliar others and deterred by their very otherness. As noted, he expressed his contempt for the lower classes, looked down on Eastern European Jews (disowning his family roots in Eastern Europe), despised the Americans, and regarded women as inferior. He admitted that he disliked psychotics, "these sick people," and confessed to being "angry at them" and seeing them as "so far from me and all that is human" (Gay, 1998, p. 559).

The impact of Freud's difficulty acknowledging the otherness and separateness of the other on his theory

The other is seen in Freudian theory as an elusive entity rather than as a unique human being with a distinct human presence and singular characteristics.

Starting in infancy, the other – at that stage, the mother figure – is perceived as an object for the projection of intrapsychic phantasies related to the satisfaction of instinctual impulses rather than as a human being in its own right with a unique personality, feelings, needs, wishes, and goals of its own, and is thus divested of its otherness and subjectivity. Relationships with the other and the involved complexities and differences of the parties to the relationship are thus excluded from the scope of discussion of Freudian theory.

The narrative of the Freudian Oedipal drama reflects the personal point of view of the narrator and his self-perception as a competitive and combative, sexually driven and physically superior male. As noted, Freud identified with valiant warriors like Hannibal while shrinking from and belittling anything and anyone that was strange to him. His discussion of female psychology, unlike that of male psychology, was superficial and lacked serious, in-depth reflection. Freud (1926) regarded women and their sexuality as "a 'dark continent' for psychology" (p. 212), an enigmatic, unexplored territory that could not be explored. Furthermore, he saw female sexuality in a negative light just because it was different from male sexuality. Aron and Starr (2013) enlarged on this point:

> Famously referring to adult female sexuality as a 'dark continent'. . . Freud equated women's sexuality with dark, uncivilized, primitive, savagery, the same qualities his society projected onto Jews, who were considered primitive, off-white, mulatto.
>
> (p. 225)

Freud's difficulty acknowledging the otherness of the other, as related to his attitude to women in general, is further reflected in the rather limited presence of the mother figure in his case studies, while the father figure was prominently featured as playing a significant role in the lives of his patients.

One may wonder why the issue of incest was likewise given center stage in the Freudian Oedipal drama. Aron and Starr (2013) attributed it to the anti-Semitic propaganda of the time, which accused Jews of being incestuous, speculating that Freud defensively sought to show that incest was a universal rather than a unique Jewish phenomenon. I would like to suggest another explanation. It may well be that Freud was sexually abused by his father or by his nanny or was witness to sexual abuse of his sisters by his father. Indications of this may be found, inter alia, in his early seduction theory of neuroses, which traced back neuroses to sexual abuse in childhood by an adult. Freud described himself as neurotic, and he apparently believed that he had been exposed to sexual abuse in his early childhood. Indeed, he explicitly said as much in one of his letters to Fliess (cited by Ferris, 1997): "Unfortunately, my own father was one of these perverts and is responsible for the hysteria of my brother (all of whose symptoms are identifications) and those of several younger sisters" (p. 135). In another reference to the issue, Freud described his nanny to Fliess as his "teacher in sexual matters" (p. 148).

Earlier, in the first of a series of letters to his best friend on fathers as seducers, written after the death of his father, Freud reported a dream he had. As related by Ferris (1997):

> In a 'nice dream' on the night after the funeral, . . . Freud was in a barber's shop, . . . where he saw a sign that read, 'You are requested to close the eyes.' Freud said it meant that one should do one's duty to the dead. Perhaps, as writers have speculated, it had something to do with closing his eyes to his father's incestuous deeds.
>
> (p. 140)

Freud's theorizing on the sexually charged relationship between little children and the adults taking care of them was apparently based on his personal experience of sexual abuse. Yet Freud subsequently dropped his original seduction theory, which presupposed sexually abusive conduct on the part of the caretaking adult, and later on focused – apparently defensively – on infantile sexuality and the sexual phantasies of the children themselves. The emphasis on sexuality as a central organizing principle of the psyche in the theory of Freud could perhaps be attributed to his own difficulty with sex. Freud himself admitted as much in a letter to a friend when he was just 39 years old and already then, "was much relieved to have left the troublesome matter of sexual life behind" (Renik, 2006, p. 151).

The clinical setup established by Freud was centered on the presence of the patient, while the analyst was supposed to serve as a tabula rasa onto which the patient was invited to project his innermost feelings, thoughts, and phantasies. The analyst was thus required to mask his own presence and maintain analytic neutrality, analytic anonymity, and analytic abstinence. This setting, whereby the patient was to lie on the analytic couch, with the analyst out of sight, ruled out the simultaneous presence of two different persons, or distinct subjects, in the analytic process. The analyzed object, that is, the patient, was not seen as a unique human being who could influence the analyst or be influenced by the analyst's presence. Rather, the analyst was cast in the authoritative, know-all position, which fitted the patient into a metaphorical bed of Sodom, depriving him of the opportunity to express a different point of view. As in the case of Dora, the patient was expected to unquestioningly accept the analyst's judgement as the living God's word, which left no place for an open dialogue or interaction between two subjects.

The psychoanalytic approach proposed and practiced by Freud reflects his difficulty in acknowledging the otherness of the other. It was adapted to his own personality and personal needs rather than to the other and to the perceptions and needs of the other. As a staunch advocate of rationality seeking to uncover the underlying unconscious truth, Freud "was especially sensitive to having knowledge withheld from him and . . . inclined to give knowledge and truth values a disproportionately exalted position" (Kohut, 1984, p. 58), albeit at the expense of empathy for his patients. His purely analytic, emotionally distant approach thus failed to offer an effective therapeutic response for those who were in need of emotional support or a close relationship with the therapist as a key component of the therapeutic process.

Donald Winnicott – Life as a comic opera

Donald Winnicott was born in Plymouth, England, on April 7, 1896, to a prosperous Methodist family. His father was a partner in the family business and a civic-minded local activist who served twice as mayor of Plymouth and was even knighted. However, due to his many activities, Donald's father did not have much time for his family. Donald's mother was a housewife. The family lived in a spacious private house surrounded by a large courtyard with a swimming pool, a tennis court, and a vegetable garden on the grounds. Donald's childhood was seemingly stable, with no apparent upheavals or traumas. Being the youngest in the family, with two sisters who were five and six years older, Donald grew up as an only child and was taken care of by several mother figures – his mother, his two sisters, his aunt who lived on the premises, and a nanny and a governess. Not much is known about his mother, yet there are various indications of her persistent depression, countered by a manic defense mechanism manifested in bursts of excitement and frenzied activity.

Donald was a well-behaved and ingratiating boy until at the age of nine, he noticed, to his dismay, that his image in the mirror was "too nice" (Rodman, 2003, p. 19). He felt that it reflected his compliance with others' expectations and the shackles put, so to speak, on his true self. In reaction, he adopted a wayward behavior, neglecting his schoolwork, using bad language, and even torturing flies, pulling off their wings. When Donald turned 13, his father decided to send him to a boarding school, where he believed the educational atmosphere would have a beneficial effect on the young adolescent. The father, who was dominant and domineering, with narcissistic characteristics, was perceived by Donald as a threatening figure, although he never explicitly admitted it. Yet as a youth and even later on, as a grown-up adult, Donald feared his father. Thus, for instance, when he planned to enroll for medicine studies after his graduation from high school, he sent his good friend Stanley Ede to inform his father of his wish, apprehensive about a negative response by his father, who expected him to join the family business. And it was only when he was over 50, following his father's death, that he dared divorce his first wife, Alice, after 26 years of a frustrating marriage. Donald was quite different from his masculine, pragmatic, unimaginative, humorless father. In fact, the dissimilarities between the two were so striking that, as Stanley observed, it was hard to believe that they were a father and son. Donald, on the other hand, was highly imaginative and creative, with an urge to express his bubbling creativity. He was fond of rhyming funny verses, toying with word games, drawing and doodling, for instance, scribbling a mouse as a signature, and so on. He felt much closer to his mother and sisters than to his father.

Displaying a keen motherly intuition, he was adept at communicating with little children and acutely aware of their needs, as remarkably reflected later on in his work as a pediatrician and psychoanalyst. Winnicott's extraordinary skill of interaction with children is touchingly illustrated in his account of the case of Diana (Winnicott, 1971):

> Diana took her small teddy bear and stuffed it into my breast pocket. . . . I suddenly put my ear to the teddy bear in my pocket and I said: 'I heard him say something!' She was very interested in this. I said: 'I think he wants someone to play with', and I told her about the woolly lamb that she would find if she looked at the other end of the room in the mess of toys under the shelf. Perhaps I had an ulterior motive which was to get the bear out of my pocket. Diana went and fetched the lamb, which was considerably bigger than the bear, and she took up my idea of friendship between the teddy bear and the lamb . . . In the play Diana decided that these two creatures were her children. . . . Then she put them sleeping together peacefully . . . She now went and fetched a lot of toys . . . On the floor around the top end of the bed she arranged the toys . . . I said: 'Oh look! you are putting on the floor around these babies' heads the dreams that they are having while they are asleep.'
>
> (pp. 44–45)

Winnicott coined and discussed at length the concept of the *good enough mother*, the ultimate caretaking figure with whom he totally identified while consistently ignoring the role of the father figure in his theory of early emotional development, with the exception of some brief references to the issue toward the end of his life. His identification with his mother was reflected, inter alia, in a slip of the pen, when he wrote her about his imminent enlistment in the army, "I wonder when *you* will really be called up" (Rodman, 2003, p. 35) [italics added]. His identification with his mother and with feminine figures, in general, was expressed even more explicitly in his comment with reference to the Jungian concept of *anima*: "For me, the anima is the part of any man that could say: I have always known I was a woman" (Winnicott, 1964, p. 451). The phrase "I have always known I was a woman" reflects Winnicott's own feelings rather than Jung's perception of the *anima* as an "inner feminine figure" that "plays a typical, or archetypical, role in the unconscious of a man" (Jung, 1961/1989, pp. 221–222). It seems that Winnicott's high-pitched voice and relatively short height for a man underscored his feminine demeanor, matching his inner leanings. In his discussion of transference in psychoanalysis, the analyst is presented as a motherly figure, the *good enough mother*, rather than as a father figure (the way the ultimate analyst was seen by Freud).

The numerous letters that Donald sent to his mother and sisters during the four years of his studies at the boarding school presented a vivid and humorous picture of his life at school. It appears that he was socially popular, the well-liked funny guy who used to amuse and entertain his friends. He played the piano, joined the school choir, took part in sports activities as a member of the rugby and cricket teams, was involved in communal projects, and so on. However, while his stay at the boarding school was conducive to his development and enjoyable in various respects, the picture he painted in his letters was no doubt too rosy. He surely had painful experiences, which he tended to deny both to himself and to others, much like his depressive mother, who adopted a manic defense as a means of evading reality. The very fact that he was sent away from home must have been a painful blow to Donald. The sharp transition from the sheltered home environment, where he was the adored precocious child, to an unfamiliar place, where he had to carve out a niche for himself in a group of peers, was most likely a tough ordeal in itself. Indeed, throughout life, whether as an adolescent or later on, as an adult, Winnicott found it difficult to separate himself from his home and family. And as observed by Clare Winnicott, his second wife (Winnicott, 1989/2018):

> Moreover, there is a sense in which the quality of his early life and his appreciation of it did in itself present him with a major problem, that of freeing himself from the family, and of establishing his own separate life and identity without sacrificing the early richness. It took him a long time to do this.
>
> (p. 10)

Judith Issroff (2005/2018), who was supervised by Winnicott, heard from him about the less rosy and more complex aspects of adaptation to boarding school life. Thus, he told her that there had been days when he was so distressed and in such deep despair that he thought of throwing himself into the cold and muddy waters of River Cam. The position taken by Winnicott against the evacuation of children during war and provocative assertion that leaving the children at risk in regions under air raid was preferable to their premature separation from home provides another indication of the immense difficulty he himself experienced when leaving home.

Upon graduation from high school, Winnicott went on to study medicine, but his studies were interrupted with the onset of World War I in 1914. At the age of 20, while still a medical trainee, Winnicott was enlisted as a medical officer and served on a Royal Navy destroyer. His military service was quite easy and nontraumatic as he was spared active participation in the battles and could use his free time to read his favorite books and listen to music. On the whole, Winnicott had a comfortable and stable life, devoid of any shattering traumas, although he did undergo a challenging period during the Second World War and suffered from a coronary heart disease later in his life. With a regular income from work and a steady financial support by his father, Winnicott did not have to struggle for economic survival, and being childless, he was spared the demanding task of raising children. Most of the time, he had housemaids at his service, taking care of routine household chores, and even a secretary who, in addition to helping him with his writings, ran errands for him, taking his car to the garage or fetching ordered books from the bookstore. No wonder then that Winnicott could preserve his childlike, lively temperament (this is, of course, not the only reason) and take a rather distant, matter-of-fact view of human evil and the horrors of war. As noted by Reeves (2004), Winnicott actually believed in "the inevitability, not to say the necessity, of war" (p. 436):

> Any lingering doubt that Winnicott did not regard war as either unnatural or inherently evil is surely dispelled by the following quotation from a little-known review he wrote of a lecture given in 1941 by a fellow analyst, J. C. Flugel, on "The Moral Paradox of Peace and War": "It is very unlikely that any investigation which sets out to find a way to end war will get far in the understanding of it. *War might turn out to be the only true integrator* (183; italics added).
>
> (p. 436)

In the following years and until the end of his life, Winnicott worked at the Paddington Green Children's Hospital in London as a pediatrician and a child psychoanalyst while also counseling parents. Unlike Freud and Kohut, who had no experience as child therapists and whose theories on psychological development in infancy were based on their psychoanalytic work with adults, Winnicott learned a lot through his direct work with infants and young children, whereby he gained valuable insights about developmental processes in early childhood. As of 1940, he served as a psychiatric consultant to the governmental evacuation scheme, deriving even more insights from his work with evacuated children in hostels during the Second World War. He discussed the issue of childcare in radio programs for mothers while carrying on his work with adults as a psychoanalyst.

At the age of 27, Winnicott married Alice, who was four years older. The childless marriage lasted 26 years. Alice was an artist, a painter, a sculptor, and ceramist, and quite a strange woman. For instance, she believed that her parrot was an incarnation of Lawrence of Arabia and used to talk with the bird. She was a reckless driver, crossing junctions heedless of red traffic lights, falling asleep while driving, or otherwise endangering herself, the passengers riding along with her, and passersby. She was highly dependent. Thus, for instance, when she had to get from London, where the couple lived, to Plymouth to sign some document in the presence of Winnicott's father, she put it off time and again, unable to do it on her own, until finally, accompanied by a friend to the train station, she went there. Her relationship with her husband lacked mutuality. While Winnicott was the supportive partner, both emotionally and functionally, his own emotional and intellectual needs remained unmet. Furthermore, their relationship was apparently platonic due to Alice's reluctance to have sex and Winnicott's own difficulties in this area. At the same time, their shared love for art and music brought them close together. In his fifth decade of life, during his work as a psychiatric consultant to the governmental evacuation scheme, Winnicott met Clare, a psychiatric social worker, who was to become his second wife, but, as noted, it was only after his father passed away several years afterward, when Winnicott was 53, that he felt free to divorce Alice and marry Clare. Unlike Alice, Clare was a strong and assertive woman, with her feet on the ground, and she played an active and vital role as a partner to Winnicott. The two shared their feelings and thoughts with each other, enjoyed spending time together on weekends, and used to exchange views and theorize about psychoanalytic issues. His years with Clare were the best Winnicott ever had, the happiest and most productive years of his life. In 1979, eight years after the death of Winnicott, Clare was awarded the Most Excellent Order of the British Empire for her work with evacuated children during the war.

Although Winnicott gradually gained prominence in the psychoanalytic community and was twice elected as president of the British Psychoanalytical Society, he remained an outsider for the most part, removed from the inner circle of the influential figures of the era. He was never interested in surrounding himself with a group of adherents or establishing himself as the leader of a clique. The psychoanalytic world was in turmoil during his years of activity, in particular, in the 1940s. Heated controversial discussions divided the British Psychoanalytical Society, with the followers of Anna Freud on the one side and the supporters of Melanie Klein on the other side. Winnicott, true to his mild temperament, was associated with the Independent or Middle Group (as it was then known) of British analysts, who allied with neither side. However, he was more deeply involved with Klein and her school, emotionally as well as on the theoretical level. Their paths crossed more than once. Klein was his supervisor over a period of five years. She referred her 27-year-old son to treatment with Winnicott and analyzed his second wife. Winnicott himself underwent analysis with Joan Riviere, who was a close colleague of Klein. In his early writings, Winnicott held a dialogue, as it were, with Kleinian concepts and seemed to agree with Klein's fundamental view of the child's destructiveness as a key element in primitive emotional development, although he saw it in a different light. For years, he sought to gain her professional recognition while making it difficult for her to grant his wish. Winnicott referred to her concepts as *subjective objects*, investing them with his own meanings and interpretations and using them in his own way. He criticized Klein for ignoring the influence of the external environment on early infantile development, condescendingly observed that training and experience as a physician (which Klein lacked) were a prerequisite for treating psychotics, and challenged her in various other ways. Yet, surprisingly, Klein, who was by nature argumentative and confrontational, adopted an accommodating and containing approach with regard to Winnicott. In fact, it was hard to be angry with Winnicott. He avoided direct confrontations as far as possible and did his best to give his interlocutor a good feeling. He was attentive, humorous, and amicable. As an analyst, Winnicott encouraged positive transference, assuming the role of the *good enough mother* who is sensitive and responsive to the patient's needs. It stands to reason, then, that his patients were no exception and similarly were unlikely to be angry with him. There was something endearingly childish about him. He was fond of playing games, including word games, particularly imagination games. He had a keen sense of humor. He liked playing music, doodling, and riding a bicycle. Like a little child, he expected Clare to admire his drawings, persistently demanding her appreciative attention, to the point of exhausting her. He used to carelessly risk himself, engaging in mischievous antics, even in old age, when he was about 70. He was caught by a policeman one day riding a bicycle with his feet up on the handlebar. On another occasion, he climbed up a tall tree next to his house to cut off its top, as it obstructed the view from his window. Life was seen by Winnicott as a comic opera, and on more than one occasion he was heard to say that "if he hadn't been a psychoanalyst he would like to have been a comic-turn in a music-hall" (Phillips, 1988/2007, p. 30). Winnicott certainly knew how to amuse others and enjoy the pleasures of life himself.

In his review of Jung's (1961/1989) *Memories, Dreams, Reflections*, Winnicott (1964) classified himself "in the category of people who in Jung's words:"

> 'always remind me of those optimistic tadpoles who bask in a puddle in the sun, in the shallowest of waters, crowding together and amiably wriggling their tails, totally unaware that the next morning the puddle will have dried up and left them stranded.'
>
> (p. 450)

This self-description by Winnicott is indicative of the manic defense he adopted in an attempt to deny, just like his mother, the gloomy reality of life. Having survived a series of heart attacks in his last years, Winnicott passed away at home following another cardiac event in 1971, at the age of 74.

Winnicott's narcissistic personality traits

On the face of it, Winnicott did not seem to be the typical narcissist. However, as noted in Chapter 3, alongside the outwardly grandiose narcissists, there is another, less conspicuous group of shy, vulnerable narcissists whose grandiosity is not openly manifested. Winnicott belonged with the latter, the characteristically more introverted, gentler, and more considerate narcissists. As described by Goldman (1993), "Winnicott was a graceful narcissist" (p. 9).

Winnicott's grandiosity

Already at the beginning of his career, Winnicott entertained fantasies of eminence and glory, as reflected in a letter to his sister written when he was just 23: "I am now practicing so that one day I shall be able to help introduce the subject [psychoanalysis] to English people so that he who runs may read" (Rodman, 2003, p. 42). Stimulated by his early aspirations of greatness, Winnicott saw himself later on as the spiritual heir of Freud in place of Jung, who lost his standing as the crown prince when he challenged Freud's drive theory and subsequently developed his own analytic psychology. Winnicott envisioned himself as the continuing son who, unlike Jung, was living up to his father's – Freud's – expectations, and hence as the one likely to rule one day the promised land of psychiatry. Winnicott shared much in common with Jung, whom he adored and with whom he identified. They were both Christians brought up in religious families and thus outstanding in the psychoanalytic community of the time, which was largely dominated by Jews (Anna Freud, Michael Balint, Melanie Klein, Heinz Hartmann, and Margaret Mahler, among others). They were both highly imaginative and artistically inclined – personal tendencies that colored and shaped their conceptualization and theorizing. Jung's theory is rich in symbols, myths, and dreams, and similarly, the writings of Winnicott highlight creativity, imagination, and life in the *potential space*, "where cultural experience is located" (Winnicott, 1971, p. 100). Winnicott's focus on the self and the expression of the authentic self brings to mind the Jungian archetype of the self and the related individuation process of synthesis of the self and self-realization. Likewise, the concept of *the false self* proposed by Winnicott is basically analogous to the Jungian *persona* archetype. Also, the female element (being) present in the male personality and the male element (doing) present in the female personality discussed by Winnicott (1971) are correspondingly suggestive of the Jungian concepts of *anima*, the "inner feminine figure . . . in the unconscious of a man," and *animus*, the "corresponding [masculine] figure in the unconscious of woman" (Jung, 1961/1989, pp. 221–222). Furthermore, Winnicott and Jung had a similar childhood experience, growing up with a depressive mother and a religiously dogmatic father as idolized, gifted only sons (Jung was an only son until the age of nine, when his sister was born, and Winnicott was the youngest in the family and the only son, with two sisters who, as noted, were his elders by five and six years, respectively). Winnicott was fascinated and, at the same time, mystified by Jung's personality and ideas. Intrigued by Jung's (1961/1989) partly autobiographical book *Memories, Dreams, Reflections,* Winnicott (1964) critically reviewed it, belittling Jung as a person and a psychoanalyst and thereby revealing his own grandiose sense of superiority. Thus, Winnicott suggested that Jung's description of his first years of life pointed to "early-childhood schizophrenia" (p. 450) and further implied that by comparison, Jung was less healthy mentally. Noteworthy in this context is a dream reported by Winnicott (1989/2018), which he had while reviewing Jung's book. The dream consisted of three parts. In the first part, the world was destroyed and Winnicott himself was destroyed along with all others. In the second part, Winnicott was the destructive agent. In the third part, Winnicott dreamed that he woke up and realized that the first two parts were a dream. Winnicott's dream calls to mind a recurrent vision recounted by Jung

(1961/1989), one of the most significant visions he had on the destruction of the world. Winnicott saw his dream as highly meaningful in that it enabled him to integrate the two split-off parts of his personality, the destroyed part and the destructive, aggressive part, and thus heal the split. This, in contrast to Jung, who, while acknowledging the split in his personality, seemed "to have no contact with his own primitive destructive impulses" and therefore never healed the split. Winnicott ascribed it "to a difficulty Jung may have had in being cared for by a depressed mother" (Winnicott, 1989/2018, p. 229) – indeed, much like Winnicott himself.

A poem written by Winnicott toward the end of his life, entitled *The Tree* (cited by Rodman, 2003, pp. 290–291), is his most explicit reference to and the clearest evidence of his mother's depression, whose "inward death" he sought to cure (the title of the poem alludes to her maiden name, Wood). An underlying theme of the poem is Winnicott's identification with Christ (Phillips, 1988/2007; Rodman, 2003), another greater-than-life figure, to whom Winnicott compared himself, nailed to the cross, carrying his own cross, trying to enliven his depressive mother (as noted by Phillips, 1988/2007, p. 29, "the Tree of the title is the Cross"). Winnicott's identification with Jesus Christ was displayed in another context, when during a meeting with Marion Milner, who was his colleague, close friend, analysand, and supervisee, he created a miniature of Christ on the cross, using matches and rubber bands. Millner interpreted it as an expression of his deep distress due to his frustrating marriage with Alice, his first wife (Rodman, 2003).

Another indication of Winnicott's grandiose self-perception, beyond his identification with illustrious figures like Jesus and Jung, was his belief that he was endowed with unique, superior abilities of therapy. Thus, he believed that in certain cases, he could bring about a major change for the better in the life of a patient in just a few psychotherapy sessions. "It is as if he felt that an ounce of Winnicott was worth a pound of pedestrian psychotherapy," a psychiatric social worker who worked with him observed (Goldman, 1993, p. 10). Furthermore, Winnicott believed that he was the only one capable of treating certain patients. In this context, Hanna Segal sarcastically commented, "from Winnicott's point of view, . . . there was only one good mother, and that was Winnicott himself" (Rodman, 2003, p. 263). In the same spirit, Orange (2011) noted, "Whether through grandiosity, hubris, generosity, or simple enthusiasm, he [Winnicott] sometimes accepted patients whom many now, and sometimes he himself in retrospect, considered seriously unwise choices" (p. 168). Thus, for instance, Winnicott chose to analyze Marion Milner, although, as noted, he had a rather complex relationship with her as her colleague, close friend, and supervisor and, moreover, as the analyst of her husband. Also, a girl who stayed for several years with Winnicott and Alice as a foster child was a patient of Milner, whom Winnicott supervised in that case too. Such blurring of boundaries was characteristic of Winnicott and directly linked to his self-perception as an omnipotent psychoanalyst. Another case in point is that of Masud Kahn, the brilliant and charismatic

Pakistani self-anointed prince who was qualified as a psychoanalyst in London but over the years became ever more aggressive and ever more blatantly unrestrained, until he was expelled from the British Psychoanalytical Society, ending up as a ruined alcoholic. Kahn was analyzed by Winnicott over more than 15 years; however, ultimately, Winnicott failed to help him (Hopkins, 1998). It seems that Winnicott was unaware of his fundamental difficulty in dealing with aggression, and hence with patients like Kahn. Furthermore, Winnicott took Kahn as a patient notwithstanding the complexity of their relationship. Kahn's spouse was also a patient of Winnicott for a time during Kahn's analysis, and Kahn himself served as editor of Winnicott's works free of charge, which could be seen as exploitation of the therapeutic relationship. Thus, once again, Winnicott displayed his disregard of boundaries, which is typical of narcissists, who perceive themselves as unbound by convention and as exempt from the rules and norms that bind "ordinary" people. Both Milner and Kahn, who closely knew Winnicott, commented on his view of himself as an omnipotent psychoanalyst. His disregard of boundaries was reflected in other ways, too, for instance, in scheduling therapy sessions contrary to acceptable psychoanalytic practices, extending session duration or setting a low-frequency schedule (thus, Winnicott met with Harry Guntrip for a prolonged session once a month during a seven-year-long analysis). Winnicott even took the liberty of having physical (nonsexual) contact with his patients. However, several months before his death, Winnicott (1984/1990) acknowledged his inflated self-perception:

> I do not need to go far to find an inflated psychotherapist. There's me. In the decade called the thirties I was learning to be a psychoanalyst, and I could feel that, with a little more training, a little more skill, and a little more luck I could move mountains by making the right interpretations at the right moment. . . . But sooner or later the process of growing smaller starts, and it's painful at first, till you get used to it.
>
> (p. 190)

Winnicott's belated acknowledgment reflects a certain moderation of his narcissism in his advanced years and a more balanced perception of his limitations.

Winnicott was basically a shy person. Yet when he was confident of his standing, he did not hesitate to take the stage and show off in his own creative and unique way. As noted, while still at boarding school, he used to amuse his classmates, clowning, playing the piano, and so on. Likewise, at the Paddington Green Children's Hospital in London, where he worked, he did not miss a chance to impress his colleagues and interlocutors with puns, witticisms, and funny or even eccentric behavior. Milner likened him to a circus performer amazing his audience with spectacular acrobatics. She actually saw him in acrobatic action when she visited him one day and was welcomed by Winnicott sliding down the banister from the upper floor, cheerfully whistling like a hyperactive child. Issroff (2005/2018) described another episode that illustrates the tactics employed by Winnicott to indirectly attract attention. At one of the Tavistock lectures delivered by a research assistant of John Bowlby, Winnicott was bored by the tedious presentation of statistical research findings collected over more than 15 years. In fact, he had serious reservations about the use of empirical and statistical research methods in the field of psychology, considering it superficial and mechanistic. He moved restlessly in his chair, rolling his eyes in annoyance, and after a while left the room, inadvertently stepping on the feet of his fellow listeners, with his finger over his lips in a 'keep quiet' gesture. Needless to say, no one could ignore his exit.

By the same token, the style Winnicott adopted in his writings reflects his obsessive need to stand out. It was important to him to put his concepts and ideas in his own idiosyncratic language, which was at times puzzling and hard to decipher and annoyed his colleagues and readers. Winnicott was well aware of this, and as he himself admitted (as cited by Rodman, 2003):

> Firstly, there are not very many creative people in the Society having ideas that are personal and original. I think that anyone who has ideas is really welcome and I always do feel in the Society that I am tolerated because I have ideas even although my method is an annoying one.
>
> (p. 176)

Hopkins (2004) quoted Milner as attributing Winnicott's insistence on his unique phraseology to his omnipotent sense of self:

> "He annoyed me, always using his own words." And she was openly contemptuous of one of his famous comments, made to Clare, that his greatest fear was that he would never have another original idea. Milner's comment about this was, "What's the big fuss he's making? It was his omnipotence that made him have that worry."
>
> (p. 242)

Winnicott's dogged adherence to his vague, abstruse, peculiar style of writing, which was incompatible with the common language used in the psychoanalytic community, could also be ascribed to his wish to achieve recognition for his unique contribution and, at the same time, traced to his need to veil his ideas and not be fully understood, triggered by his schizoid anxiety of intrusion by others (his schizoidism is discussed in more detail hereinafter).

The way Winnicott referred to his mortality is characteristic, in a sense, of the omnipotent narcissistic experience, which denies the finality of life and thereby, one's limitations as a human being. It is noteworthy that Winnicott chose to open the autobiography that he started to write in his last years under the title *Not Less Than Everything* with a few lines from T. S. Eliot's *Four Quartets* contemplating "the end," seen by Eliot as "a beginning." Reflecting on his own approaching death, Winnicott followed with a seemingly paradoxical wish, "Oh God! May I be alive when I die" (Winnicott, 1989/2018, pp. 3–4). His prayer may be interpreted as an omnipotent denial of reality, of the finality of life, of nonbeing, of the place where we no longer exist.

Winnicott's vulnerable, inferior, dissociated sense of self

Winnicott's feelings of inferiority were indirectly reflected in various ways. Throughout his life, Winnicott sought to express his authentic self. At the same time, he felt that he had to conceal the less appealing aspects of the self, that is, internalized aspects of the self perceived as inferior and devalued. As noted, already as a nine-year-old child, Winnicott tried to shake off his ingratiating image as "too nice" and adopt a defiant, willful manner that would express his true, authentic self, the way he saw it then. As an only son born several years after two sisters, he was presumably expected to fulfill the role of the long-awaited male child. Yet, brought up by "multiple mothers," Winnicott identified primarily with the feminine figures who had taken care of him and later chose a career path in therapy, working with children, like his mother and sisters, most of his life. This was apparently a blow to his father, who hoped to see his son following in his footsteps and joining the family business, as befitted a man. "My father was there to kill and be killed, but it is probably true that in the early years he left me too much to all my mothers," Winnicott recalled (Phillips, 1988/2007, p. 27). He felt let down and rejected by his father, all the more so when he was sent away to boarding school at the age of 13. It seems that the feeling that he disappointed his father played a major part in Winnicott's vulnerable, inferior sense of self. Could it also be his fragile masculinity, frowned on by society, that contributed to his feelings of imperfection? As he told Clare, already as a young child, he felt "uncomfortable with his girl-self" (the "too nice" self) and thus sought to be more of a boy, an unruly, aggressive, "hating" boy (Orange, 2011, p. 156, citing Neve, 1992). Winnicott's lifelong difficulties in sexual function no doubt further undermined his self-esteem as a man. Indeed, Clare expressed her disappointment that Winnicott was not masculine nor resolute enough (Rodman, 2003). Beyond the issue of manhood and masculinity, Winnicott's self-deprecation was evident in his relationship with Clare, on whom he was deeply dependent and without whom he felt worthless. As related by Rodman, "He would awaken in the night and tell her, 'I'm potty about you, do you know that?'" (p. 104). In a letter to Clare from 1946 cited by Rodman, Winnicott wrote, "When I am cut off from you I feel paralysed for all action and originality" (p. 91).

Winnicott's feelings of inferiority were also reflected in his relationship with James Strachey, with whom he had his first analysis. Winnicott felt illiterate and uncultured compared to Strachey, whom he highly regarded as a man of culture. This is noteworthy since for Winnicott, culture was "the only medium for self-realization" (Phillips, 1988/2007, p. 119) and a rich cultural life, the apex of self-development.

It is also of note in this context that Winnicott was concerned about moving out of West London, where his practice was based, fearing that "no one would refer patients to him anymore" (Rodman, 2003, p. 104), although at the time, he was already well-established professionally and enjoyed widespread acclaim. His self-doubt and insecurity were thus further displayed.

Winnicott's split personality

Winnicott himself acknowledged his dissociated sense of self. Yet he believed that he had managed to heal the split. Winnicott (1989/2018) explicitly discussed his split personality with reference to the three-partite dream of the destruction of the world described earlier, in which he was first destroyed along with the rest, then took part in the destruction as a destructive agent, and finally realized that it was a dream – an experience that contributed to the integration of his personality. While he held back "an immense amount of detail that is personal and that can be ignored" (p. 228), so that the exact nature of his personality split and of each split-off self-state remained obscure, it may be assumed, based on his theory, that he was speaking of the split between the true self and the false self. The concept of *the true self* coined by Winnicott denotes the grandiose sense of self that evolves and thrives when an omnipotent experience of the self is enabled. It is an aggressive, vital, and vibrant aspect or "core" of the personality that is essentially self-sufficient, "never communicates with the world of perceived objects" (Winnicott, 1965, p. 187), and "must never be affected by external reality" (p. 133). By contrast, *the false self* denotes the weak, imperfect, submissive, and compliant aspect of the personality, devastated by external reality. Margaret Little (as cited by Rodman, 2003) noted with reference to Winnicott's dualism of the true self and false self that he was a modest, unassuming person and, at the same time, had a grandiose, omnipotent sense of self that had a defensive function and served as a compensation for his feelings of inferiority and insecurity.

The impact of Winnicott's grandiosity on his theory

Narcissistic grandiosity is the axis around which the Winnicottian theory revolves. Winnicott drew a direct line between a grandiose sense of self, on the one hand, and creativity and mental health, on the other hand. He saw grandiosity as the source and foundation of an authentic, meaningful life, in infancy as well as in adulthood. Infantile narcissism is innate, according to Winnicott. In this earliest stage of primary narcissism, the infant is self-absorbed and perceives himself as omnipotent. This illusion of omnipotence, that is, of unlimited magic power, is contingent on consistent maintenance and cultivation by a *good enough mother*. When the mother adapts and caters to the needs of her baby without fail, feeding him when he is hungry, adjusting the room temperature to make him feel comfortable, providing appropriate stimulation whenever required, and so on, she fosters the infant's illusion of omnipotence, the illusion that he himself, like a god, creates and shapes the world around him to suit his needs and desires.

Winnicott believed that this type of relationship between mother and infant should be adopted in psychoanalytic therapy to provide the patient with the facilitating, responsive environment essential to personal development and growth, which he probably lacked as a child. In this context, Mitchell and Black (1995/2016) noted:

> In his work with more disturbed patients, Winnicott made every effort to shape the treatment around their spontaneously arising needs. Even setting regular times for sessions creates an artificial, external structure to which the patient needs to adapt, like an infant fed according to schedule rather than on demand. So Winnicott would try to provide sessions on demand. He told of one young woman he would watch for from behind the curtains. Timing was crucial. As she approached his front door and raised her hand to knock, he would open the door, as if her wish for him in fact had created him.
>
> (p. 133)

Winnicott (1965) believed that timing was also critical for the interpretations offered by the analyst in the therapeutic setting and that the patient should be given the feeling that he rather than the analyst had come up with the interpretation since "if we make the interpretation out of our own cleverness and experience then the patient must refuse it or destroy it" (p. 182). However, my clinical experience of over 30 years shows that in many cases, the patient actually appreciates the interpretation provided by the analyst, of which he might not have been aware. It should be noted, though, that narcissistic patients, to whom Winnicott apparently referred and with whom he identified, find it difficult to accept the analyst's interpretations as such acceptance could be seen by them as indicative of their imperfection and their need for the other.

The mental health criteria established by Winnicott, supporting his superior self-perception, further reflect his grandiosity. It is thus no chance that the key criterion for mental health proposed by Winnicott highlighted the capacity for creative playing, taking place in the *potential space*, as an expression of the true, authentic self. As noted, Winnicott was highly imaginative and creative, with a penchant for playfulness, and enjoyed playing music, drawing, and squiggling, which he also used as a therapeutic technique. One of the overarching goals he set for therapy was thus empowering the patient to realize his potential for playing. At the same time, Winnicott chose to ignore pathological aspects of the personality that could reflect his own personality failures. Thus, for instance, he empathized with children diagnosed as antisocial and rather than considering their behavior indicative of a clinical disorder, the way Bowlby saw it (Issroff, 2005/2018), Winnicott attributed their antisocial tendency to deprivation in early childhood and saw their behavior as a healthy manifestation of their hope to regain what they had been deprived of in their early formative years (Winnicott, 1984/1990).

Winnicott's schizoidism

The life history of Winnicott shows that he was rarely emotionally involved in his interpersonal relationships. This could be attributed to his schizoid personality traits (McWilliams, 2006) as well as to his shy, vulnerable narcissism (as contrasted with grandiose narcissism). Winnicott's 26-year-long marriage with Alice was largely devoid of intimacy. It was a platonic relationship, more like that between a parent and a child than between partners in a couple relationship. Alice was an eccentric, bruised woman-child who found it difficult to deal with routine, everyday tasks. It seems that Winnicott projected onto Alice his dependency needs, which he denied for years, while undertaking the role of the responsible adult. Throughout those years, he entertained a feeling of self-sufficiency, living in a schizoid glass bubble or cocoon, which was gradually cracked during his second marriage to Clare. The nature of his relationship with Clare as well as other aspects of his life discussed hereinafter point to the moderation of his narcissism with the years, which enabled his involvement in a more mutual relationship, a closer, more intimate, and more fulfilling relationship. In this context, his underlying dependency needs, repressed during his frustrating marriage to Alice, emerged in full force, and he became so dependent on Clare that he did not believe he could create anything of value without her.

Winnicott's avoidance of too close interpersonal relationships was manifested in his relations with James Strachey and Joan Riviere, with whom he was in analysis for years. Winnicott's first analysis, with Strachey, lasted ten years. Winnicott saw in Strachey, who was his senior by nine years, an elder brother – and, in certain respects, an object of envy – rather than a father figure. It seems that Winnicott chose a relatively young analyst to avoid dealing with his complex, unresolved feelings toward his father. Be that as it may, Winnicott described his relationship with Strachey as anything but close or warm and the attitude of Strachey as "cold-blooded" (Rodman, 2003, p. 75). Riviere, who, as noted, was a friend and a colleague of Klein, was Winnicott's second analyst. His seven-year-long analysis with Riviere was likewise characterized by a distant and cold relationship. Furthermore, it was highly conflictual and antagonistic, so much so that Riviere wondered whether she should carry on with the analysis. Winnicott, for his part, went as far as to say that if he had learned anything from the analysis with Riviere, it was how not to go about it. Besides, Winnicott had unsettled financial issues with both analysts, bargained with them, skipped payments as if unintentionally, and as Strachey suspected, was not telling the truth about his due payments. Given that Winnicott was well-off and even financially generous in certain cases, his conduct in the matter could be seen as passive-aggressive and, furthermore, it raises doubts about his capacity for intimacy, even with long-standing associates like Strachey and Riviere.

On the whole, the relationships established by Winnicott were asymmetrical. For the most part, he assumed the role of the supporting, coaching therapist and thereby maintained his narcissistic sense of superiority. With the exception of his relationship with Clare later on in his life, Winnicott stuck to an emotionally distant, self-sufficient position in his interpersonal relationships while denying and suppressing his dependency needs. Milner, a psychoanalyst in her own right, and, as noted, Winnicott's analysand, supervisee, and close friend, recounted an illustrative episode (Hopkins, 2004). At a certain point in her analysis with Winnicott, she realized that she had to choose between being his analysand and being his supervisee in the case of the foster girl who was taken care of by Winnicott and Alice. It was a painful choice for her, and she burst into tears when she decided to give up analysis. Winnicott was quite surprised at her emotional response. Milner saw his reaction as a gross denial of the intense emotional relationship evolving in the therapeutic setting. As shown in this and other cases, Winnicott failed to acknowledge the significance of close emotional relationships per se, irrespective of the fulfillment of needs.

The work practices and writing style adopted by Winnicott provide further indication of his schizoid personality. Winnicott preferred to work alone, formulating his ideas without interacting with colleagues or associates. And as noted, his abstruse style was meant to keep his readers at a distance and his writings not fully comprehensible. Mitchell (2014/2023) described the style of Winnicott as "poetic and elusive" (p. 80). It seems that Winnicott used his stylistic elusiveness as a defense against intrusion by the outside world, displaying the characteristic schizoid anxiety of intrusion.

Winnicott's mother passed away when he was about 30. However, my review of his works and correspondence has revealed no reference to the way he dealt with the loss. Likewise, no expression of grief or mourning over the death of his father years later could be found in Winnicott's writings, and apparently, not by chance. The little that is known about his emotional reaction to the loss of his parents has been written by his biographers, which points to the defensive emotional distance that he kept even from those close to him.

The impact of Winnicott's schizoidism on his theory

According to Winnicott's model of psychological development, in early infancy the infant is self-absorbed and focused exclusively on himself and his needs, existing in a state of primary narcissism, oblivious of any object relations. While with time, the infant gradually becomes aware of his mother as a separate object, her presence has significance for the infant only insofar as she provides basic functions that enable his ego development (holding, providing a nonintrusive environment, responding to the infant's spontaneous gestures, etc.) rather than as a unique object of emotional attachment. It is noteworthy that Winnicott, who was greatly influenced by Klein, disagreed with her view of primary object relations and adopted instead the notion of primary narcissism proposed by Freud and advocated by his daughter Anna. Yet Winnicott is considered – unjustly so, in my opinion – an object relations theorist. In fact, rather than focusing on object relations per se, Winnicott's theory revolves around the self, and to the extent that he referred to object relations, it was in the narrow context of the mother-infant relationship, that is, with regard to maternal care, which is essential to self-development and self-growth.

Two of Winnicott's seminal papers on emotional development, *The Capacity to be Alone* and *Communicating and Not Communicating* (Winnicott, 1965), highlight his view of "the permanent isolation of the individual" (p. 189), which glorifies the schizoid tendency. Inter alia, Winnicott wrote:

> I suggest that in health there is a core to the personality that corresponds to the true self of the split personality; I suggest that this core never communicates with the world of perceived objects, and that the individual person knows that it must never be communicated with or be influenced by external reality. This is my main point, the point of thought which is the centre of an intellectual world and of my paper. Although healthy persons communicate and enjoy communicating, the other fact is equally true, that *each individual is an isolate, permanently non-communicating, permanently unknown, in fact unfound.*
>
> (p. 187)

Winnicott further elaborated on "the threat to the isolated core" of the individual, which he deemed "sacred," noting, "Rape, and being eaten by cannibals, these are mere bagatelles as compared with the violation of the self's core, the alteration of the self's central elements by communication seeping through the defences" (p. 187). The observations made by Winnicott in this context are no doubt of interest as they shed light on the inner personal space, where the individual would rather not give others a foothold. However, Winnicott took it a bit too far when he likened the communication seeping through to the isolated core to no less than "rape" or "being eaten by cannibals." The extreme language he used seems to reflect his excessive schizoid anxiety of intrusion of the self by the other. In the same spirit, Guntrip (1968/1992) raised doubts about Winnicott's "dubious proposition," maintaining that as long as the infant experienced a positive relationship with his environment, no such permanently withdrawn, isolated core of the self, "cut off and defended against all intrusion of the outer world" (p. 4276), should develop.

The ambivalence displayed by Winnicott with regard to close intimate interpersonal relationships was variously reflected in his writings. Thus, Winnicott (1965) discussed the ability to establish relationships with objects as part of the maturational process and as indicative of emotional development, noting, "A further development is in the capacity for object relationships. Here the infant changes from a relationship to a subjectively conceived object to a relationship to an object objectively perceived" (p. 45). However, in the same breath Winnicott qualified his argument and emphasized the importance of keeping a distance from others and preserving the "isolation of the individual" or, in other words, the "isolation of the true self" (p. 46). Enumerating the stages of maturation, Winnicott reiterated the importance of the isolation of the individual. Thus, the third stage "of personal childhood development" was, according to Winnicott, "The development of a capacity to make relationships with objects in spite of the fact that in one sense, and an important sense, the individual is an isolated phenomenon and defends this isolation at all costs" (p. 68).

The distinction made by Winnicott (1971) between *object-relating* and *object-usage* provides another indication of his ambivalence regarding close interpersonal relationships. The concept of *object-relating,* which would seem to signify a mature and mutual relationship with a separate object, denotes, in Winnicott's terminology, a relationship with a *subjective object* that has no existence in itself except as a provider of the infant's needs. Similarly and contrary to what might have been understood, Winnicott coined the corresponding concept of *object-usage,* which has a negative connotation of an exploitative and functional relationship with a part-object, to indicate a healthy and mature relationship with an objectively perceived separate object. It appears that Winnicott's choice of such confusing terminology reflects his own ambivalence regarding the intrinsic emotional need for the other and for a close relationship with the other.

No wonder then that Winnicott did not consider love an inherent emotion that develops naturally in the context of the relationship with the parental figure. In contrast to Balint (1968/2013), who discussed primary love as the earliest level of object relationship, Winnicott (1971) saw love as a secondary product of the infant-mother relationship that develops following a phase of aggressive dynamics instigated by the infant and that allows for love to emerge only after the mother survives the infant's aggression, is thus perceived as an external object, and can therefore be loved by the infant. However, as argued by Rudnytsky (1991), the presumption adopted by Winnicott, drawing heavily on Klein, that love relationships must have an irreducible core of aggression is not empirically supported. Winnicott's discussion of love invariably involved reference to negative feelings of hate, aggression, or guilt, reflecting his difficulty in submitting to the intimacy of love. Rather than dealing with close emotional relationships and their significance, his writings on interpersonal relationships, love relationships (Winnicott, 1988), or the psychology of separation and mourning processes (Winnicott, 1984/1990) are replete with instinctual terminology. Concepts such as the Oedipal complex, penis envy, and pre-genital and genital impulses are discussed at length in that context, and object relations are seen as originating in aggressive and sexual impulses, while intimacy and emotional attachment are only marginally considered. Although Winnicott discarded, albeit implicitly, the Freudian drive theory when discussing the self, his treatment of the issue of interpersonal relationships is based on the classical theory of instinctual drives. His dread of intimacy was manifested, inter alia, in his dismissal of the importance of the infant's unique personal relationship with the mother. In this context, Winnicott (1988) observed:

> It is here if at all that the technique rather than a personal relationship is important, so that in these matters there is a relatively smaller necessity for the mother to be the person in charge. In other words, if the technique of infant care is good, the matter of who it is that employs the technique is not so important.
>
> (p. 156)

Elaborating on the issue, Winnicott further noted:

> In the psychology of the individual, however, there is an important aspect of relationships in which it can be said that in the most intimate contact there is a lack of contact so that essentially each individual retains absolute isolation always and for ever.
>
> (p. 157)

Likewise, Winnicott (1984/1990) played down the significance of emotional attachment in his discussion of the psychology of separation and loss and grief processes, specifically in situations of loss of a parent or separation from a parent. Thus, there is no real consideration of the emotional agony caused by the loss or separation and no reference to the hole in the child's soul, to the missed love, or to the painful longing. The discussion focuses on the child's feelings of hate and aggression toward the deserting object and on the child's capacity or incapacity for mourning as a measure of mental health, as illustrated in the following passage, "illness results not from loss itself but from the occurrence of loss at a stage in the child's or infant's emotional development when a mature reaction to loss cannot take place. The immature ego cannot mourn" (p. 113). Elsewhere in *Deprivation and Delinquency*, Winnicott noted with reference to the reaction of a two-year-old child to his mother's long absence upon reuniting with her:

> Investigation showed that Eddie could not easily meet his mother again because in the time of separation from her he had hated her without being able to get from her presence and smile the reassurance that she could remain alive and friendly in spite of his hate.
>
> (p. 17)

Discussing the impact of the home environment on emotional development, Winnicott (1988) stated, "The death of parents is easier for children to stand or to recover from than the complications arising out of emotional difficulties between the parents" (p. 153).

Another illuminating case of parental loss and separation described by Winnicott (1989/2018) concerns a child who, on his eleventh birthday, lost his father in a drowning accident, which the child miraculously survived. Referred to analysis by Winnicott eight months after the tragic event, the child showed psychosomatic symptoms and seemingly slight paranoid reactions. Yet rather than focusing on processing the loss of the father and on the child's relationship with the father, Winnicott chose to devote the best part of the ten-session analysis, which was conducted over a long period of more than a year (and complemented by four sessions with the mother), to an early childhood separation experience of the child, when at the age of a year and a half, he had to cope with the absence of his mother, who was hospitalized for a few weeks due to a surgical procedure. The handling of the case by Winnicott points to his difficulty dealing with son-father relationships and, at the same time, is illustrative of his difficulty acknowledging the significance of emotional attachment to and the loss of an attachment figure even at a later stage in life.

Likewise, Winnicott (1989/2018) criticized the interpretation offered by Bowlby in the case of *A Two-Year-Old Goes to Hospital*. While Bowlby saw the distress of the little girl as reflecting her longing for and mourning of the loss of her mother, who (in line with the then common practices) was not allowed to visit her at hospital, Winnicott maintained that mourning was contingent on personal maturity and could only take place at a more advanced stage of development. Furthermore, Winnicott seemed to underestimate the significance of the separation from the mother, noting that "the trauma when a child is separated from the mother is often not the loss of the mother but the loss of the thing that I call a transitional object" (p. 431). That is, he saw the loss of the *transitional object* as more significant than the separation from the real-life mother. Similarly, discussing the "separating-out of the not-me from the me," Winnicott (1971) minimized the implication of the separation from the significant attachment figure, citing the *potential space* (in analogy to the *transitional object*) as a substitute for that significant human figure. In this context Winnicott noted:

> At the same time, however, it can be said that separation is avoided by the filling in of the potential space with creative playing, with the use of symbols, and with all that eventually adds up to a cultural life.
>
> (p. 109)

However, is separation indeed avoided? It could perhaps be mitigated. The use of the word "avoided" once again highlights the minimization of the significance of both the separation from and dependence on the real-life parental figure.

Finally, Winnicott dealt primarily with anxieties related to the disintegration of the self and the intrusion of the self by the other and less so with the anxiety of abandonment by a loved object, which further indicates his focus on the defense of the self or, as he put it, the isolated core of the individual, and failure to duly consider the significance of close interpersonal relationships per se.

Winnicott's difficulty acknowledging the otherness and separateness of the other

As shown, Winnicott expected the other to serve as his extension, so to speak, much like Freud and Kohut. However, unlike either Freud or Kohut, Winnicott simultaneously manifested in his interpersonal relationships the very opposite position of self-deprecation. He seemed to have difficulty in maintaining a mutual relationship where the partners to the relationship recognize each other and communicate with each other as separate subjects (Benjamin, 1999). His self-deprecation, bordering on masochism, was evident throughout his years-long spousal relationship with Alice. Undertaking the role of the supporting partner, Winnicott apparently did not expect Alice to show consideration of his needs. To a large extent, he sacrificed himself for her, giving up his otherness and separateness, which exacted a heavy mental toll on him. It is noteworthy, however, that the self-denial and masochism associated with the role of the devoted caregiver, savior, and martyr serve a narcissistic function, enhancing the grandiose self-experience and sustaining an omnipotent narcissistic position (Ronningstam, 2005). The same omnipotent role of a savior-martyr was assumed by Winnicott in his childhood with respect to his depressive mother, whom he felt obliged "to enliven . . . to cure her inward death," as he wrote in his previously cited poem *The Tree* (Phillips, 1988/2007; Rodman, 2003).

The blurring of boundaries shown by Winnicott with regard to his own otherness and separateness was reflected, inter alia, in his choice of life partners, who resembled him in many respects. Alice, his first wife, was an artistically inclined, unrealistic, and rather strange woman, quite like Winnicott, for whom creativity was central to life and whose eccentric behavior was displayed every so often (Issroff, 2005/2018). And as further noted, they were both sexually inhibited. Winnicott's relationship with Clare, his second wife, although more mature, was largely based on likeness rather than on individuality. They shared intellectual and professional areas of interest as well as a preference for playful leisure activities. And they were both childless. While, as noted, Clare was a strong and assertive woman, she seamlessly adapted to Winnicott's lifestyle, sparing him the need to cope with her otherness. It is not surprising then that, as she related, they enjoyed an essentially harmonious relationship. Yet in their marriage, Winnicott often assumed the role of the sole subject, demanding exclusive attention, consideration, and support, straining Clare to the limit. The nature of their relationship and her role in the relationship are aptly illustrated in Clare's account of a letter she received from Winnicott in 1950 "in which he described his love for her as being in part the love he had for his 'transitional object,' a girl doll" (Rodman, 2003):

> One aspect of their relationship therefore was that in her "good-enough mothering" she made herself available to be re-created in the image of his desires and needs in a way that she not only did not challenge but actively encouraged. She also provided him with near-perfect "mirroring" as can be seen in her comments on how she was shown all of his "squiggle" productions . . . "There were his *endless* squiggle drawings which were part of his daily routine . . . If I was away for a night he would send a drawing through the post for me to receive in the morning, because my part in all this was to enjoy and appreciate his productions, which I certainly did, but sometimes I could wish that there were not quite so many of them."
>
> (pp. 103–104)

It appears then that although Clare found it difficult to deal with Winnicott's persistent demands, she could not possibly ignore his wishes and expectations of her and thus involuntarily donned the image of the *good enough mother* or, alternately, the *transitional object* conceived by Winnicott and applied in that context for his own use.

In the same way, Winnicott expected Klein to acknowledge and appreciate his theoretical contributions, showing a childish disregard for the other's subjective feelings and needs. As noted, Winnicott took the liberty of borrowing from Klein and modifying her concepts at will as his own *subjective objects*. Furthermore, he challenged her theoretical frame of reference and superciliously referred to her lack of medical qualifications (which he deemed a prerequisite for treating psychotics). Nonetheless, he expected her to survive his attacks, as it were, and fulfill his wishes. In his imagined relationship with Klein, Winnicott saw himself as the sole subject – occupying the same position at the center of the universe as the infant in his theory of the parent-infant relationship, where the presence of the mother as a unique human being with feelings and wishes of her own is played down to the point of near irrelevance.

On the whole, Winnicott did not show much interest in interpersonal relationships unless he played a vital role in the relationship. He was mainly self-centered, focusing on his work, writings, and attempts to draw applause from an appreciative audience, whether in everyday situations or on more formal occasions (e.g., lectures). The significant relationships in his life were often characterized by a blurring of boundaries between the personal and the professional, which put him in the authoritative, know-all position and freed him from the need to cope with the otherness and separateness of his partners in the relationship (e.g., the need to consider divergent views, to deal with the exposure of vulnerable aspects, or to handle ambivalent, complex emotions). His relationships with Marion Milner and Masud Khan, who trusted and adored him as their supervisor and analyst (as well as the analyst of their spouses) and who were his colleagues and friends, are two prominent cases in point.

Winnicott's preference to work on his own rather than collaborate with others is indicative of his difficulty in dealing with divergent ideas proposed by others. By keeping a distance from others, he was able to maintain the narcissistic illusion of a unique existence and a perfect, omnipotent sense of self that was not overshadowed by the actual presence or talents of others, who were delegated to serve as extras in the imaginary show revolving around him. Furthermore, Winnicott tended to ignore the contribution of other theorists, and to the extent that he drew on the work of others, he used their concepts as he deemed fit, as he himself explicitly admitted. Thus, when presenting a paper to the British Psychoanalytical Society in 1945, he said (Phillips, 1988/2007):

> I shall not first give a historical survey and show the development of my ideas from the theories of others . . . What happens is that I gather this and that, here and there, settle down to clinical experience, form my own theories, and then, last of all, interest myself to see where I stole what.
>
> (p. 16)

His manifested disdain for the ideas of others, which he saw as mere fragmentary notions, insignificant in themselves, provides another indication of his disregard for the feelings of others. And even when he found where he "stole what," he often failed to give credit where credit was due, taking all the credit for himself. At the same time, Winnicott was highly sensitive about others borrowing from him without crediting him. Thus, for instance, as related by Issroff (2005/2018), "Brett Kahr . . . had seen in the New York archive Winnicott's copy of Bowlby's book that he had reviewed in 1953 . . . and Winnicott had noted in several places that Bowlby had not cited his work" (p. 58).

Be that as it may, Winnicott generally refrained from reading the psychoanalytic works of other theorists for fear of discovering that they had anything of value to contribute to his theory, which could threaten his narcissistic sense of self-perfection. For instance, as related by Goldman (1993, citing Rodman, 1992), "Winnicott was reluctant to read the works of Ferenczi, lest he discover that he had actually stolen ideas from him" (p. 5). Winnicott did not even bother to delve deeply into the writings of Freud (Kahr & Bechdel, 2016), not to mention other theorists and writers. As further related by Goldman (1993, citing Khan, 1975), when Khan urged Winnicott to read Lionel Trilling's *Freud and the Crisis of Our Culture*, Winnicott rejected Khan's suggestion:

> It's no use, Masud, asking me to read anything. If it bores me I shall fall asleep in the middle of the first page, and if it interests me I will start re-writing it by the end of that page.
>
> (pp. 4–5)

Indeed, rewriting others' concepts was a habit of Winnicott, as shown in his treatment of Klein's concepts, which, as noted, he regarded as *subjective objects*, as he himself put it. Hanna Segal sharply criticized Winnicott for taking Klein's theory, recasting it in his own vision, using it to his own ends, and assuming full credit for the end product. (Rodman, 2003). In response to similar criticism by Balint regarding Winnicott's claim to exclusive originality, Winnicott expressed regret in his last years for his failure to recognize the contribution of others toward the development of his own theory (Rudnytsky, 1991).

It is noteworthy that in the case of Freud, Winnicott adopted a glorifying and, at the same time, guarded approach. He seemed to project his father's image onto Freud and in both cases chose to avoid direct confrontation. While, as noted, Winnicott hardly read Freud's writings, he masked the highly significant differences between them and presented his own theory, which was innovative and revolutionary in various respects, as merely another layer of conceptualization building on Freud's theory. The position adopted by Winnicott with respect to Freud points to his difficulty acknowledging the option of dissimilarity and otherness, which could be stressful in a sense, but which does not necessarily challenge or play down the other, and which may even be inspiring and stimulating.

The impact of Winnicott's difficulty acknowledging the otherness and separateness of the other on his theory

"There is no such thing as an infant," Winnicott (1965, p. 39) observed, highlighting the inseparability not only of the infant but also of the mother (Ogden, 1986/1990), whose subjective existence should thus blend into that of her infant and become irrelevant. From the Winnicottian perspective, in the early stages of development, the infant is the sole subject entitled to attention, and his needs and desires take center stage. A premature awareness of separateness would thus be a negative and traumatic experience for the infant rather than a normal, primary developmental experience, as maintained by Klein, Fairbairn, and Kernberg, among others. Hence, the mother in Winnicott's model is required to be totally attentive to the infant's needs, to meet all his physical and emotional needs, and to mirror his emotions while minimizing her presence, and, in fact, ignoring herself and her own needs and thereby providing the infant with the nonintrusive holding environment that is essential to his early development. However, such requirements seem not only unfair to the mother but also unrealistic, as they disregard the deep impact the mother has on the infant as a unique human being with a life of her own. Furthermore, while interacting with and caring for her infant, the mother has other relationships to maintain and other concerns to attend to that involve other children she may have; her couple relationship, which is likely to be affected by pregnancy and birth; her relationship with her parents; and her own anxieties, wishes, moods, and changing self-image. So, at what stage and in what context does awareness of the otherness and separateness of the mother emerge as per

Winnicott? His theoretical position on the issue is not clear-cut. On the one hand, Winnicott described the significant journey taken by the infant on his way toward independence and separation while distancing himself from the mother in the process (along the lines of the model proposed by Mahler). On the other hand, he failed to address the complexity of the infant's evolving relationship with the mother and its associated aspect of otherness, as the infant gradually perceives the mother as a separate object. Winnicott first tackled the issue of relationships with a separate other at a rather late stage in his life and theorizing, when he proposed the concept of the *object-mother*, that is, the mother eventually perceived by the infant as a separate object, and the corresponding concept of the *environment-mother* (Winnicott, 1965), whose sole purpose is to provide a facilitating environment for the development and growth of the self while she stays in the background as a vital yet unnoticed presence, like oxygen for life. As noted, according to Winnicott, the discovery of the mother as a separate object follows episodes of infantile aggression, which the mother survives without taking revenge, being destroyed, or moving away from the infant, who thus realizes that his influence on the mother is limited since she is a separate human being and, as such, can be loved by him. However, Winnicott did not elaborate on the infant's rich and complex relationship with the *object-mother*. It seems that he felt closer to the *environment-mother*, whose elusive presence is essential to infantile development. The internalization of the *environment-mother* was seen by Winnicott as highly significant and as crucial to the development of a healthy true self. At the same time, the internalization of the *object-mother* was hardly discussed in his writings (the issue was enlarged on by Kernberg, Klein, and Ogden, among others), although the *object-mother* and other significant attachment figures playing a key role in early infancy have a distinct and identifiable impact on the self-perception of the individual later on in life. Apparently, the option of any major transformation of the true self due to the formation of external object representations that are internalized and integrated as intrapsychic object representations by the infant was inacceptable to Winnicott, which is not surprising considering his schizoid anxiety of intrusion. And to the extent that he referred to identification with the other, it was in the context of the false self rather than the true self.

Winnicott saw the relationship between analyst and patient as analogous to the relationship between mother and infant and thus believed that the patient should be given the opportunity to experience the inseparability of the early infancy relationship in the therapeutic setting. In this context, Winnicott (1971) observed, "Psychotherapy is not making clever and apt interpretations; by and large it is a long-term giving the patient back what the patient brings" (p. 117). In other words, Winnicott advised the analyst to minimize his otherness and adapt himself as far as possible to the patient and to the way the patient perceived and interpreted his experiences in the therapeutic setting. It seems that it reflected Winnicott's own need for self-expression that is not restrained by the presence or intrusion of the other.

Winnicott's difficulty acknowledging the otherness and separateness of the other was also clearly reflected in the way he understood and interpreted the human psyche, which he saw through the lens of his own personal experience and mental world. For Winnicott, the self – the key concept of his theory – was at the core of emotional life, and the capacity for expression of the authentic self, a prime goal and a prerequisite for mental health. As shown, Winnicott himself went through a tortuous journey on the way to the realization of his own true self, starting in childhood, when at the age of nine, he decided that he was no longer interested in being the well-behaved and ingratiating boy reflected in the mirror, whose spontaneity and aggressiveness were inhibited. Winnicott believed that the expression of the authentic self was no less significant for others and hence a universal human quest. However, this is not the case for everyone. For some, expression of the authentic self may be naturally realized (and often involves inconsiderate or even aggressive behavior), while others may not necessarily consider it an overarching goal. Furthermore, it is not universally considered a valuable or desirable goal. As noted in Chapter 1, there are cultures that value communality above individual self-realization (Orange, 2011; Rubin, 1998). But did not the members of such ancient traditional cultures enjoy a significant life just because they did not consider the individual self and self-realization their top priority? And are not the members of contemporary non-Western communities that highlight group solidarity and commitment living a significant and mentally healthy life? The answer seems to be clear.

Winnicott's focus on the realization of the true self is closely associated with his basically positive view of aggression as the manifestation of vitality and authenticity and as reflecting a mature perception of reality (Winnicott, 1965, 1971). As noted, Winnicott found it difficult to deal with aggression, whether his or others'. An episode related by his analysand Margaret Little (1990) is just one of many cases illustrative of his reaction to aggression:

> In one early session with D. W. I felt in utter despair of ever getting him to understand anything. . . Then I thought of throwing out all his books, but finally I attacked and smashed a large vase filled with white lilac, and I trampled on it. In a flash he was gone from the room, but he came back just before the end of the hour. Finding me clearing up the mess he said, "I might have expected you to do that [clear up? or smash?] but later." Next day an exact replica had replaced the vase and the lilac, and a few days later he explained that I had destroyed something that he valued. Neither of us ever referred to it again, which seems odd to me now.
> (p. 43)

Winnicott's largely positive view of aggression as the manifestation of vitality, authenticity, growth, creativity, and maturity rather than as the destructive and devastating expression of pathology reflects his blindness to its pernicious and ruinous consequences. In fact, Winnicott found positive aspects even in war, notwithstanding the horrors, traumas, and human suffering that it caused, of which he seemed to be oblivious, as reflected in his declaration "we fight to exist" and further shown in his "surprisingly even-handed statement" that "If we fight to exist, we do not thereby claim to be better than our enemies" (Reeves, 2004, p. 435).

There are other examples of Winnicott's generalization and universalization of his own personal experience and mental world. Thus, for instance, he attached great importance to the capacity to be alone (Winnicott, 1965) as well as to the ability to play and create (Winnicott, 1971) – abilities that distinguished him personally – as central to the human psyche. He proposed a regressive reconstructive clinical practice that encouraged the patient to reenact and reexperience his infantile dependency, apparently, since he himself was in need of such corrective emotional experience as a means of expressing his own repressed infantile dependency needs, which for years he projected onto others. And he rarely dealt with sexuality or the development of a sexual identity, which was not surprising given his difficulties in this area.

Heinz Kohut – Illusive images

Heinz (Wolf Hirsch) Kohut was born on May 3, 1913, in Vienna, the capital of the Austro-Hungarian Empire, the only child of his Jewish parents. His father, Felix, was an aspiring pianist at the time, and his mother, Else, an artistically inclined singer. Kohut was just a little over a year old when his father enlisted in the Austro-Hungarian army at the outbreak of World War I in 1914. Throughout the war years, his father served on the front line and eventually fell into captivity of the Allied Powers in Italy. Kohut moved with his mother to her parents' home in a village outside Vienna for the duration of the war, and except for short visits during those years, Kohut did not see his father until the age of five. When his father finally returned from the war in 1918, the family moved back home to Vienna. However, following the long separation and in the wake of the war events, the relationship between the parents fell apart, and although they continued to share the same household, their paths parted as a couple.

The father, a lively and spirited man before the war, became a quiet, reserved, and sad person, traumatized by his war experiences. He did not return to playing the piano and finally gave up his musical aspirations and moved into business. As a child, Kohut was seldom witness to his father's former joie de vivre. On one of those rare occasions, when his father took him for a ski vacation, he had the opportunity to see his father as he had once been, a vivacious man, full of charm, enchanting the visitors at the ski resort with his piano playing at the bar, flirting with the waitresses, and delighting the onlookers with fascinating stories. But as noted, it was a rare event. Most of the time, Kohut experienced his father as emotionally distant and even critical of him. Thus, his father, who was an artist at heart, found it difficult at first to appreciate Kohut's interest in science. Later on, their relationship warmed, but just as they were getting closer together, when Kohut was about 24, his father fell ill with leukemia and passed away within six months. The loss of his father prompted Kohut to seek psychotherapeutic treatment for the first time in his life.

Kohut's mother, a creative and dominant, yet unstable woman, raised her son as if he were her extension, an inseparable part of herself. She did not let him express wishes of his own or form relationships with others. It seems that the absence of Kohut's father, actual absence during the war and emotional absence following the war, as well as the fact that Kohut was an only child and thus the center of his mother's attention made it even worse for him. Until the age of five, Kohut slept in his mother's bed and even after his father returned home, he slept in his parents' room, in a separate bed, for another three years. When, at the age of eight, Kohut moved into a room of his own, his mother did not allow him to close the door. In fact, she was so intrusive as to check his stools on a daily basis and obsessively clean blackheads on his face throughout his childhood while, as Kohut felt, showing no real interest in him. Furthermore, his mother did not send him to school until the fifth grade. As an alternative, she hired private tutors to take care of his education, ignoring his need for socializing with other children. His loneliness remained a constant companion during the following school years. He seldom invited friends home and spent his leisure time engaging in solitary sports (rowing, cycling, jogging, skiing), piano playing, and reading fine literature. Even on vacations he was usually sent alone. As a youth, Kohut enjoyed going to the opera, attending concerts, watching theater shows, visiting art galleries, and hanging out in the Viennese cafés, often accompanied by Ernst Morawetz, one of the mentors hired by Kohut's mother. Morawetz, in his twenties at the time, was the first close friend Kohut ever had. Spending time together, they used to hold stimulating intellectual discussions. Kohut looked up to Morawetz and felt happy with him. At a certain point, their emotional intimacy evolved into a sexual relationship.

At the age of 19, Kohut began his medical studies at the University of Vienna. During the six years of his studies, he stayed at his mother's home. While he had no significant intimate relationship with the other gender during that period, he became more socially involved. In the course of his internship in Paris, he met Jacques Palaci, a Jewish student of medicine from Turkey, with whom he established a lifelong friendship. Kohut was invited to visit Palaci at his parents' home in Istanbul, where he was genially hosted for a couple of weeks. However, Palaci felt that his hospitality was not reciprocated. Kohut, who got used to being alone, only rarely invited Palaci to stay with him in Vienna, and on the few occasions that Palaci visited him, he was met with an atmosphere of mystery, emptiness, and "solitude," with "no feeling of life there," as Palaci described it (Strozier, 2001, p. 48). Kohut's mother was not present to welcome him. Instead, the two, host and guest, were served by a maid in uniform. Notwithstanding their close friendship, there seemed to be an invisible wall dividing them, set up by Kohut and veiling significant aspects of his life. Thus, Palaci not only never met Kohut's mother but was not even told that Kohut's father had passed away. The reserve and secretiveness displayed by Kohut in his relationship with Palaci were typical of him and manifest as a recurring pattern throughout his life.

Kohut was 25 when in March 1938, Nazi troops marched into Austria and Hitler announced its annexation to Germany. The Nazi occupation of Vienna "left Kohut with the feeling, as he put it, of a 'crumbling universe'" (Strozier, 2001, p. 55). "That summer a series of anti-Semitic laws were passed. . . All Jewish bank accounts were frozen" (p. 56). Jews were banned from the theaters, the museums, the concert halls, and the opera, which were an inseparable part of Kohut's life and cultural identity. Signs reading "No Dogs or Jews Allowed" were posted in front of the coffeehouses that he used to frequent. "Overnight he became radically devalued and a persona non grata" (p. 55). Thus, practically against his will, Kohut was faced with his Jewishness, which he sought to disown all through his life, even before the Nazi takeover of Vienna (as discussed in more detail hereinafter). For instance, when Kohut visited Palaci in Istanbul, he presented himself in a way that baffled his Jewish hosts, leaving them in doubt about his Jewish identity. As related by Strozier (2001), "He [Kohut] seemed to be Jewish, had a Jewish name, and had Jewish sensibilities. But in all the discussions of politics and culture he acted as a non-Jew and put himself outside of the frame of reference of Jewish concerns" (p. 48). Even Palaci, his close friend, was not sure if he could take at face value Kohut's disclosure that he was Jewish on both sides and for years doubted whether what Kohut had told him was really true. Be that as it may, Kohut, like Freud before him, had no choice but to escape the Nazi regime. Leaving behind the collapsing Viennese world, Kohut moved first to a refugee camp in England, and when he received a visa to the United States about a year later, he crossed the Atlantic in February 1940 and settled in Chicago. His mother, who could not make it out of Austria with him, joined him the following year in Chicago, where she lived not far from him for the rest of her life.

Once settled in his new country, Kohut started medical residency in neurology. Having been certified in neurology but uninterested in this field, he went on to specialize in psychiatry. In 1942, Kohut applied for admission to the Chicago Institute for Psychoanalysis but was rejected. The reason for the rejection has remained unclear. Paul Ornstein, who was one of Kohut's disciples and his partner in the development of self psychology, suggested that "what got in the way for Kohut was his narcissism" (Strozier, 2001, p. 80). Yet Kohut managed to find a way around and, following several attempts, was eventually admitted to this highly regarded institute. In 1950, he officially became an analyst and three years later, a training and supervising analyst as well as a faculty member at the institute.

As far as known, Kohut had only one significant romantic relationship before his marriage, with a young woman named Barbara Bryant, who was ten years younger (he was 30 and she was 20 when they met). However, after a year and a half, Kohut abruptly broke off with Bryant. At the age of 35 he married Elizabeth Meyer, a 36-year-old social worker. Described as a shy and reserved woman, Elizabeth was content to stay in the shadow of her dominant husband. The couple had one child, a son, who was named Thomas August after both Thomas Mann, the novelist adored by Kohut, and August Aichhorn, with whom Kohut began psychoanalysis in Vienna following the death of his father. Kohut had a rather complex relationship with his only son. While he no doubt loved Thomas and deeply cared for him, he was often at odds with him, whether over the table manners of young Thomas or about red-hot political issues as Thomas grew up and unlike his self-centered, single-minded father, who was focused on psychoanalysis, became involved in social activism, taking part in protest rallies, hunger strikes, and the like. The message conveyed by Kohut to his adolescent son when he was away at a summer camp reflected Kohut's view on the way to cope with difficulties and the need to hide one's vulnerability: "Don't show it too much if you are out of sorts or a little homesick but keep your chin up and your spirits high" (Strozier, 2001, p. 165).

With time, Kohut carved a niche for himself in the Chicago psychoanalytic community. Following a decade of activity in the American Psychoanalytic Association in various roles, he reached the top of the organization, serving as president-elect of the association from 1962 to 1963 and as its president from 1964 to 1965. His personal charm and charisma apparently paved his way up to this senior position. Kohut was always looking impeccable, elegantly and formally dressed in a suit and tie, his feet clad in custom-made shoes. Ernest Wolf, who was a student and a follower of Kohut, recounted that once, when he was waiting with some other candidates for the elevator at the top floor of the Chicago Institute for Psychoanalysis, a "'youngish man, well dressed, of very serious mien' with a Germanic accent, whom he did not then know, came up to the group and told them that if they were traveling to the ground level it was all right to use the elevator. If however, they were simply going to the floor below where there were additional classrooms, they should not tie up the elevator but rather walk" (Strozier, 2001, p. 108). Wolf was taken aback by Kohut, "who seemed so ascetic and disciplined, so Teutonic and commanding" (Siegel, 1996, p. 8).

As an analyst, though, Kohut displayed empathy, responsiveness, and sensitivity. His remarkable skills in the therapeutic setting as well as a supervisor impressed his colleagues. Arnold Goldberg, one of Kohut's younger followers, said that he had never met anyone who was in analysis with Kohut who did not adore him. At the same time, Kohut himself "felt he had a better overall success rate in supervision than in his own practice, in which he often lost patients 'because of my own extreme sensitivities'" (Strozier, 2001, p. 361).

Kohut was a man of habits and, much like Freud, had a regular daily routine. He used to get up at 6:30 in the morning, do some sports, and then work throughout the day. In the evening, following the family dinner, he liked to listen to music and read books and took the time to handle his correspondence before retiring for a night's sleep around 2 a.m. Along with his intensive professional life as an analyst, supervisor, lecturer, and theorist, Kohut appreciated the cultural milieu. He enjoyed spending time with friends in upscale restaurants, visiting museums, attending classical music or jazz concerts, and going to the opera.

Over the years, Kohut drifted away from mainstream psychoanalysis and gradually developed his own ideas, initially focusing on the issue of narcissism and its treatment in the context of classical psychoanalysis and, later on, formulating a whole new theory – the theory of self psychology. Offering an alternative to classical psychoanalytic theory, Kohut boldly challenged the fundamental concepts and tenets of Freudian psychoanalysis (the Oedipal complex, the instinctual drives, etc.). His betrayal, so to speak, of the mainstream psychoanalytic school was unacceptable to his peers, the old guard of the psychoanalytic community, and he was increasingly ostracized. It should be noted that Kohut had been regarded for years as one of the pillars of the international psychoanalytic movement and as the prospective successor of Heinz Hartmann, the undisputed leader of the movement at the time, so that his deviation from traditional psychoanalysis was seen as all the more outrageous. Anna Freud, who had held Kohut in high esteem and used to like him, subsequently distanced herself from him. His books were harshly criticized, and he was removed from the centers of power in the psychoanalytic movement.

At the age of 56, Kohut established a discussion group along the lines of Freud's Psychological Wednesday Circle, gathering around him younger analysts who were intrigued by his ideas and helped him to develop his theory of self psychology, among them Marian and Paul Tolpin, Ernest Wolf, Michael Basch, Paul Ornstein, and Arnold Goldberg. The group carried on his legacy after his death, expanded on his theory pushing the theoretical envelope, and continued to develop the self psychology movement and its institutions. Yet while Kohut was adored by his young colleagues, some of them felt that he was not attentive enough to their needs nor duly appreciative of their individual contribution. Thus, Kohut could call any of the group members at inconvenient times, late at night or during dinner, to discuss trivial matters. And although he drew on their ideas, he failed to acknowledge and credit the unique input of each member to the formulation of his theory, giving rise to feelings of bitterness and resentment in the group.

When Kohut was 59, his mother passed away. Although upset by her presence, he had taken care to keep in touch with her on an almost daily basis, talking with her on the phone or meeting her, and at least once a week he invited her for dinner at his place. But all in all, she seemed to manage quite well on her own. After emigrating to the United States, she opened a small clothes shop, and in her spare time, she dabbled in painting for fun. She had several love affairs and, by and large, made the most of her life. However, in her last years, her health failed, and she experienced psychotic paranoid ideation. Curiously, her mental condition came as a relief to Kohut. Indeed, it was a liberating experience as he realized that of the two of them, she was the insane one, as he had suspected all those years. And he could thus understand his father, his desertion of his wife, and his consequent abandonment of his son.

A year before the death of his mother, Kohut was diagnosed with lymphoma, and for the remaining ten years of his life he struggled with the incapacitating disease and with some other comorbidities. As noted by Strozier (2001), "It would be difficult to overstate the impact that cancer had on Kohut. It shattered his personal myth of invincibility" (p. 232). Kohut experienced the cancer as something shameful, as another issue that he had to hide or lie about. "'My father,' says Thomas Kohut, 'was very intolerant of weaknesses on his part'" (p. 233). Kohut passed away at the age of 68, several days after delivering a lecture at a self psychology conference. He was drained and pale, and knowing that this was his farewell lecture, he gravely said, as many in the large audience began to cry, "I'm quite sure that this will be the last self psychology meeting that I will attend" (p. 377).

Kohut's narcissistic personality traits

There are quite a few indications of Kohut's narcissistic personality, first and foremost, his 1979 article *The Two Analyses of Mr Z*, where Kohut (1991/2011) diagnosed Mr. Z. as a narcissist, apparently molding him in his own image. Indeed, the article is believed to be autobiographical, although Kohut himself never admitted it. While Mr. Z. is presented in the case study as the analysand of Kohut, his family background and formative life events are remarkably similar to those of Kohut himself. As argued by Strozier (2001), "It seems as true as one can ever hope to know that Kohut is the subject of Mr. Z" (p. 315). Furthermore, as observed by Thomas, the narcissism of his father, "especially in public . . . was embarrassing and painful" and both he and his mother often urged Kohut to "stop being so narcissistic." According to Thomas, Kohut was aware of his narcissism and when he "was feeling good, he could acknowledge the criticism," but admitted, "I can't help myself" (p. 167). Also, as noted, Ornstein cited Kohut's narcissism as the apparent reason for the repeated rejection of his application for admission to the Chicago Institute for Psychoanalysis. Strozier, who personally knew Kohut and, as his biographer, studied in depth the life story and personality of Kohut, wrote about him, "He often enraged people or hurt them badly with his intense narcissism, but the rest he charmed as if by magic with his zest for everything" (p. 12).

Kohut's grandiosity

"Kohut had always been grandiose," Strozier (2001) stated (p. 316). Kohut's grandiosity was manifested in various ways, for instance, in his deep identification with and adoration of Freud. Kohut, like Freud, grew up in Vienna and escaped the city after its occupation by the Nazi regime in

1938. Following in the footsteps of Freud, Kohut went through a similar education and career path, studying medicine, specializing in neurology, and shifting to psychiatry and psychoanalysis. As Strozier further observed, "Perhaps Kohut's academic half year abroad at some level was also a modeling of himself after the young Freud, who left Vienna in the 1880s for Paris" (p. 46). Even at a later stage in his career, when he was developing his self psychology theory, challenging Freudian drive theory, Kohut sought to emulate Freud and as noted, established a discussion group comprising disciples and followers of his own, modeled on Freud's Wednesday Circle. Kohut recalled the departure of Freud from Vienna in June 1938 as a defining moment when, in a sense, Freud passed the torch on to him. The farewell scene on the train station platform was a deeply moving event for Kohut, so much so that he used to tell over and over again how, when tipping his hat in greeting, Freud cordially took off his hat and waved back at him. It is also noteworthy that when writing *The Restoration of the Self*, Kohut (1977) insisted on dividing it into seven chapters (including the *Epilogue*), in a format corresponding to that of Freud's (1913) *The Interpretation of Dreams*, as related by Natalie Altman, who was hired by Kohut to edit his manuscript. She added that Kohut had once told her that "the structure was intended to copy God and the seven days of creation" and as noted by Strozier (2001), "She was not sure if he was joking" (p. 281).

Citing Anthony Storr's study of gurus, Strozier (2001) observed that the childhood isolation, introversion, and narcissism shaping the development of a guru were characteristic of Kohut in his early years and that the typical charisma of a guru, which attracted adherents and devotees, distinguished Kohut later on in life. Indeed, the charismatic personality of Kohut cast a spell on many and drew a massive following. Strozier cited Thomas as observing that his father tended to dominate the scene wherever and whenever possible and that "it was very hard to share the stage with him . . . he had to be number one and the center of everybody's attention" (p. 167).

Kohut's relationships with those close to him were clearly asymmetrical. Almost invariably, he assumed the role of the wise, all-knowing, all-powerful partner while the other was in the position of an admirer, disciple, or counselee. Thus, in his relationship with Barbara Bryant, who was ten years younger, Kohut played the role of the experienced wise teacher by virtue of both his age and professional standing. A similar pattern characterized his relationship with his wife Elizabeth, who willingly left the stage to her illustrious husband, adapted to his needs, and catered to his every whim. Robert Wadsworth, Kohut's closest lifelong friend, was described by Thomas as a self-effacing, submissive person who was "happy to have my father dominate him . . . [He] ceded the stage . . . and was part of the audience" (Strozier, 2001, p. 70). Wadsworth himself acknowledged his submissiveness in a letter to a common friend, Siegmund Levarie, noting, "I have very little confidence in my ability, or my fitness, to play a part in any other life, but I hope you will try to keep a place for me in yours" (p. 69).

Kohut, for his part, displayed a condescending attitude toward others, including family members and close friends and associates, seeking to highlight his own superiority. It seems that no one was spared his arrogance, not even his best friends, as illustrated in the following episodes related by Strozier (2001). Thus, when visiting Jay McCormick, who was at the time one of his closest friends, Kohut used to throw his hat on one of two delicate and quite expensive vases received by the McCormicks as a wedding present, implicitly indicating that he thought the vases were in bad taste. On other occasions, Kohut could be deliberately disdainful toward the guests at a lunch or a dinner party, and when he discovered that no one spoke German, he would embarrass the attendees by reading out whole passages from Goethe. Likewise, David Terman, a loyal follower of Kohut and his supervisee for nearly four years, was derided by Kohut for his supposedly bad French accent, although Terman had perfect command of the language.

Kohut felt unbound by generally accepted standards of behavior, displaying the typically narcissistic grandiose sense of entitlement and disregard of the rules and norms that bind the common people. Thus, as noted, he took the liberty of calling his colleagues and disciples whenever he felt like it, heedless of the inconvenience it caused. He did not think twice about asking a former analysand to look for a car that he was interested in buying at a discount. And he felt entitled to advise patients and supervisees alike to get married or get a divorce or to tell them how and where they should spend their leisure time or which restaurants they should visit when on vacation. It is particularly noteworthy that in the case study of Mr. Z. (who, as noted, is believed to be Kohut himself), Kohut discussed the "insatiable narcissistic demands" of Mr. Z. "and his arrogant feelings of 'entitlement'" (Kohut, 1991/2011, p. 5). Kohut's absolute sense of entitlement and related views on issues of morality and integrity were reflected, inter alia, in his observation (as cited by Strozier, 2001) regarding the habit of Beethoven – another admired role model of Kohut – to fraudulently sell his manuscripts to several publishers simultaneously:

> "I would not be surprised," Kohut wrote Siegmund Levarie, "if a thorough investigation of such acts . . . would point up a higher morality, e.g. that, in order to protect and support his creative self, Beethoven considered the question of morality or immorality in the usual sense as irrelevant, just as a revolutionary might consider a murder in the service of his idealized cause as a moral act."
>
> (p. 242)

And as noted by Strozier, "Genius, in other words, marches to its own unique ethical drumbeat" (p. 242).

Kohut's vulnerable, inferior, dissociated sense of self

Kohut's vulnerable, inferior sense of self was reflected in his relentless efforts to hide significant aspects of his life that he perceived as flawed, inferior, and thus shameful – notably, his Jewish origins – and maintain a façade of perfection reflecting a superior sense of self, the perfect self that he imagined himself to be. Kohut apparently associated his Jewishness with belittling anti-Semitic stereotypes, internalizing the anti-Semitic ideology of the era, which was prevalent even before the war (Aron & Starr, 2013). It could also be that his mother's negative attitude about Judaism and fascination with Christianity had to do with his rejection of his Jewish identity. Be that as it may, throughout life, while still living in Vienna as well as after fleeing the Nazi-occupied city, Kohut was evasive about his Jewish identity. As noted, even his close friend Jacques Palaci remained uncertain for years as to Kohut's Jewishness. At times, Kohut flatly denied his Jewish origins, while on other occasions he gave vague or partial answers when asked about it. Thus, he would mumble something incoherently or counter with "Who is a Jew, anyway?" when confronted with his Jewishness. Or he would say that his father was a Jew, but his mother was a Christian (although she was a Jew by birth, whether or not she was confirmed as a Christian). Furthermore, Kohut refrained from referring to Jews as such and avoided telling Jewish jokes or admitting that he understood such jokes. He gave the impression that he knew nothing about Jewish culture or tradition. Thus, for instance, he once asked Wadsworth to explore the Jewish custom of circumcision as if he had not the faintest inkling of what it was all about, although he himself was circumcised. In his interaction with Jewish patients, supervisees, and colleagues, Kohut never mentioned his Jewish origins. Peter Barglow, a European Jewish immigrant who was in analysis with Kohut for several years, thought that he was a Christian. Michael Basch, another Jewish patient of Kohut and, later on, his colleague and a theorist in his own right, was hurt when at a dinner party, Kohut expressed surprise at his knowledge of German, although Kohut was well aware of his background as the son of Jewish émigrés from Germany who had come to the United States escaping the Nazi regime. Anna Ornstein, a Holocaust survivor and a member of Kohut's inner circle together with her husband, Paul Ornstein, felt actually betrayed when she realized that she could not discuss with Kohut anything that had to do with Judaism and the Jewish experience, in general, or his Jewishness, in particular. The following episode, related by Paul Ornstein (as cited by Strozier, 2001), is illustrative of Kohut's blatant rejection of his Jewish identity. The two once went to a kosher deli, and knowing that it was kosher, Kohut deliberately ordered a ham and cheese sandwich along with a glass of milk. When politely told that his order was unacceptable, Kohut blew up and loudly insisted on getting his order. His need to hide his Jewish identity was so deep that even his son, Thomas, was unaware of his father's Jewish origins while he was still alive. Thus, Thomas recalled that his father had told him about his close to a year-long stay at the refugee camp in England, his first stop after escaping Vienna en route to the United States, describing it as a harsh experience, mainly because all others in the camp "had an identity. They were Jewish. He was not. He was Viennese . . . he didn't have that" identity (Strozier, 2001, p. 116).

The issue of homosexuality was apparently another source of Kohut's sense of imperfection and lack of self-acceptance. As far as known, as an adolescent, Kohut had a prolonged homosexual relationship with his mentor, Ernst Morawetz, but it is not known for certain whether he had any such relationships as an adult. It was rumored that Kohut had a sexual relationship with his closest friend Robert Wadsworth, who looked effeminate and was generally believed to be a homosexual. Whether or not the rumors had a basis in fact, it should be noted that in those days, homosexuality was not considered a normal sexual activity but rather a shameful aberration that should be concealed (which, to a lesser degree, is still the case even today).

Kohut was also secretive about other aspects of his life. Thus, apparently ashamed of his mother, he never introduced her to his friends and associates. As noted, Jacques Palaci, his close friend from their days as students of medicine, who spent time together with Kohut in Vienna, was invited to visit him just a few times and, even then, was not given the chance to meet Kohut's mother, while Kohut was warmly hosted by Palaci's parents at their home in Istanbul. Likewise, Barbara Bryant, with whom Kohut had his first significant romantic relationship, which was intensively carried on for about a year and a half, was not introduced to Kohut's mother, who lived nearby and was visited by Kohut almost daily. When one day Bryant came across Kohut and his mother at a hotel restaurant, where Bryant met with a friend for a Sunday dinner, she realized that not only was she never introduced to Kohut's mother, but she had also never been mentioned by him as his romantic partner, and even on that occasion, Kohut said nothing to indicate the nature of their relationship. Similarly, Kohut's longtime friend Jay McCormick and his wife Peggy, who lived at the time in the same Chicago neighborhood, never met Kohut's mother. Once, driving with Kohut, Peggy was dumbfounded, as she later told Strozier (2001), when Kohut offhandedly mentioned that they had just passed by his mother's clothes shop but was unwilling to say more about it, then or afterward, clearly indicating that he would rather not talk about his mother. McCormick never met Kohut's closest friend Wadsworth either, although Wadsworth was usually invited to join the Kohuts on festive family dinners and eventually became a regular at their place. Apparently, Kohut felt uneasy about Wadsworth's effeminate appearance and strange mannerisms and chose not to introduce him to his friend. This and other episodes related by Strozier show how important it was to Kohut to always display a perfect image.

As noted, Kohut was equally evasive about his cancer, from which he suffered in the last decade of his life and which he sought to hide from friends and family alike. As related by Thomas in this context, his father could not tolerate weaknesses on his part. Indeed, it was not only the debilitating impact of the disease that Kohut found difficult to accept. He was unable to acknowledge any weakness or imperfection, whether real or imagined, in any sphere of his life. Shame, consciously or unconsciously experienced, seemed to be an ever-present companion of Kohut, reflecting his enduring sense of vulnerability and inferiority and accounting for his ever-present need to identify with an imagined flawless self and present an impressive façade of perfection, veiling those aspects of his life and personality perceived by him as less appealing or desirable.

Kohut's split personality

"His psychological style, one might say, was highly dissociated," Strozier (2001) observed with reference to Kohut's "deeply conflicted and split-off" attitude about and denial of his Jewish identity (p. 39). Aron and Starr (2013) similarly suggested that the way Kohut dealt with his Jewishness indicated a "vertical splitting" of the personality, linking it to his deep shame and even "self-hatred" regarding his Jewish origins:

> In our view, Kohut was Tragic Man, his life and theory dominated by intense shame and its dissociation. Kohut's central contribution, the study of narcissism, may be understood as having its origins in Kohut's deep feelings of shame and self-hatred regarding his Jewishness and the vertical splitting and dissociation of this aspect of his religious identity. (p. 57)

Thomas Kohut was likewise aware of his father's dissociative experience, although he did not use the exact term 'split personality' to characterize it. Thus, when visiting Vienna with his father after the war, Thomas discovered a completely different person than the one he knew, a more relaxed and vital man. Thomas later related that his father shared with him his experience of life in parallel in two worlds – the old world of his treasured prewar Vienna and the new world of America, where he had to build his life anew as a displaced refugee.

Another indication of Kohut's dissociative experience was provided by Kohut himself (1991/2011) in the case study of Mr. Z. (who, as noted, is believed to have been molded in Kohut's own image). Kohut described Mr. Z. as experiencing himself "in two different, separate ways," so that "his personality established a vertical split" (p. 46), where one part of the self remained attached to and intertwined with the mother and, as such, was experienced as grandiose, while the other dissociated part of the self maintained a bond, remote as it might have been, with an idealized father, which ultimately enabled Mr. Z. to detach himself from his mother and form a healthy and independent male self. Kohut saw this personality split, or "vertical split" – discussed in the case study of Mr. Z. as well as in the analysis of Mr. X. (Kohut, 1977) – as typical of the narcissistic personality and hence of himself as a narcissist. Kohut traced the vertical split to early childhood, a point on which I agree with him. Yet it may well be that having been uprooted from his homeland and cultural milieu and forced to abandon his former life in Vienna and start a whole new life across the ocean, his inherent personality split further deepened.

The impact of Kohut's grandiosity on his theory

Most theorists and researchers believe that narcissism is a manifestation of pathological and defensive aspects of the personality (Afek, 2018; Diamond et al., 2022; Bromberg, 2009; Kernberg, 1975; McWilliams, 2011; Modell, 1975; Rosenfeld, 1964; Symington, 1993). Since Kohut actually, if not explicitly, saw himself as a narcissist, he chose to characterize narcissism as a normal phenomenon that, moreover, could potentially undergo transformations and develop into more advanced, mature, and sublime forms such as creativity, empathy, the capacity to contemplate the finality of life, humor, wisdom, and cosmic narcissism. The view of narcissism as pathological was dismissed by Kohut as based on cultural prejudice. His theory of narcissism thus served him as a statement of defense, as it were, that is, as a shield against acknowledging the pathological aspects of his personality, and thereby preserved his superior sense of self. It is notable that when discussing the capacity to contemplate and acknowledge the finality of life, Kohut (1966) seemed to totally identify with "the great" endowed with this sublime ability:

> The great who have achieved the outlook on life to which the Romans referred as living *sub specie aeternitatis* do not display resignation and hopelessness but a quiet pride which is often coupled with mild disdain of the rabble which, without being able to delight in the variety of experiences which life has to offer, is yet afraid of death and trembles at its approach.
>
> (p. 265)

Kohut's apparent identification with the enlightened "great" while setting himself apart from the ignorant "rabble" echoes Freud's condescending view of the uncultured "miserable rabble."

Narcissism is manifested in early childhood as a grandiose self-experience, which is, according to Kohut (and likewise maintained by Winnicott), a foundational experience that is essential to the development of a healthy, cohesive, and vital self. Kohut believed that the primary role of the parental figures (*selfobjects*, as he put it) was to foster this experience of grandiosity – by allowing the child to idealize them and perceive them as superior and omnipotent as well as by mirroring his own superiority and omnipotence. It seems that Kohut attached so much importance to the experience of grandiosity since it was so dominant in his own life. Thus, while the concept of mirroring proposed by Kohut has been interpreted by some as encompassing all self-aspects of the child (as suggested by Winnicott), my review of Kohut's writings indicates that Kohut discussed mirroring primarily in the limited context of cultivating a grandiose sense of self – this, through the mirroring of affects, needs, and qualities related to high self-esteem, pride in one's achievements, outstanding abilities, feelings of superiority, and so on. At the same time, mirroring is rarely discussed in his writings with reference to personality traits, behavior patterns, affects, needs, or wishes that are not directly related to grandiosity or self-esteem, for instance, a sense of humor, impulsiveness, pragmatism, dependency, neatness, various emotions (sadness, fear, envy), likeness to a family member ('You are the spitting image of your mother.'), and so on. There is ample evidence of Kohut's focus on the mirroring of narcissistic grandiosity. The following are just a couple of illustrative instances.

In the analysis of Mr. M., Kohut (1977) sought to trace the origin of his patient's interrelated disturbances, and in this context he observed:

> The first one was indeed a manifestation of Mr. M.'s primary structural defect; it was genetically related to the failure of his mother's self-object function as a mirror for the child's healthy exhibitionism. . . The genetic matrix of the primary defect – stunted development of the grandiose-exhibitionistic aspects of the self – was insufficient mirroring from the side of the mother.
>
> (p. 7)

Discussing the psychoanalytic techniques that proved effective in the case of Mr. M., Kohut noted that the first was "working-through processes in the area concerned with the insufficient mirroring responses of maternal self-objects, i.e., by gradual integration into his personality of his grandiose-exhibitionistic urges" (p. 14).

In his last, posthumously published book *How Does Analysis Cure?* Kohut (1984) discussed the distinction between mirroring, idealization, and twinship. To illustrate the point, Kohut described a situation where "a friend puts his hand on our shoulder when we are troubled." This symbolic gesture was seen by Kohut as an instance of mirroring when it signified for us "approval, an expression of confidence in our innate power and in our resilience; it would constitute an expression of admiration for us even in our present state of disturbance" (pp. 198-199). It should be noted that the need for twinship was originally regarded by Kohut (1971/2009) as coinciding with the need for mirroring, and it was only at a later stage that he elaborated on his theory and defined the need for twinship as a distinct need (Kohut, 1984). The need for twinship is the need to feel similar to others in behavior, appearance, manner of speaking, and so on (displayed, for instance, when a girl imitates her mother, dressing, talking, or conducting herself like her), or to belong to a group of people who hold similar views and values, who are of the same ethnic origin or age, and the like. The need for twinship is clearly manifested in adolescence, when teenagers adopt a conspicuously similar style of speech or clothing. Yet Kohut associated the need for twinship with a sense of self-competence, that is, with the aspect of the self related to one's perceived skills and talents, which could be attributed to his biased perception and interpretation of reality through the lens of narcissistic notions of potency and self-worth, manifest even at that later stage of his life.[1] It could be concluded then that Kohut saw the self essentially in terms of narcissistic mental content and the sense of grandiosity and omnipotence as its core aspect, as aptly captured in his observation, "we now conceive of the self as consisting of three major constituents (the pole of ambitions, the pole of ideals, and the intermediate area of talents and skills)" (Kohut, 1984, p. 192). This limited view of reality is typical of the way narcissists perceive themselves and judge others – through the narrow prism of the experience of potency and self-worth, in light of issues of success or failure, capacity and superiority or incompetence and inferiority, self-realization, and so on. Indeed, Kohut's concept of narcissism and notion of the self seem to overlap, as discussed at length in my article on Kohut's theory of self psychology and pathological narcissism (Afek, 2019). While mental processes and mental content related to talents, skills, and self-worth or to the quest for an ideal self-image constitute an inseparable part of the self, other, no less significant processes come into play in the development of the self, for instance, separation and individuation processes (involving questions such as 'Am I like or rather unlike my parents?' 'Is it okay to feel angry with or estranged from my parents?' 'And what does it say about me?' 'Would I be able to manage on my own later on in life?'), internalization of parental images as intrapsychic object representations or as different self-states (thus, identification with the internalized object representation of the mother would inspire one to act and experience the world just like her), and development of a sexual identity and its implications for the perception of family roles and ultimately for the perception of the self.

The psychoanalytic therapeutic process proposed by Kohut is intended to encourage the unfolding of *selfobject* transferences, following the early stages of infantile development and focusing on infantile grandiosity. The unmet narcissistic needs of the patient (mirroring, idealization, and twinship) are supposed to be answered through *selfobject* transferences that would enable a gradual process of self-development, whereby archaic narcissism undergoes transformation and evolves into mature, healthy narcissism.

Kohut's schizoidism

In the evidently autobiographical case study of Mr. Z., Kohut (1991/2011) portrayed Mr. Z., and hence himself, as a person for whom "the area of interpersonal relationships would never play the dominant role in his life that it does for the majority of people" (p. 50). John Gedo, one of the brilliant members of Kohut's discussion group, described him as indifferent to others and aloof. This detached attitude could be traced back to Kohut's loneliness in the formative years of his childhood and youth. As noted, he was not sent to school until the fifth grade and thus was denied the opportunity to socialize with peers. He remained socially isolated during his school years, when he rarely invited friends home and mostly engaged in solitary leisure activities. His relationships with his parents were equally cold and distant, marked by hostility toward his mother and idealization of his father, who was physically absent during the war years of Kohut's early childhood and emotionally absent for years afterward. The early death of his father when Kohut was about

24, just as their relationship got closer, left Kohut with a sense of emptiness, and, as noted, prompted him to seek psychotherapeutic treatment for the first time in his life (Strozier, 2001). It is noteworthy that the social isolation that weighed down on Kohut for so long was cited by him as one of the triggers for Mr. Z.'s initial application for psychoanalysis (Kohut, 1991/2011).

Kohut displayed a detached attitude and a lack of interest in the other as a separate object even in his significant relationships as an adult. This was true for his discussion group colleagues and partners to the development of his self psychology theory, whom he saw as just a means to an end rather than as unique individuals worthy of his personal attention. It was also true for his relationship with his wife Elizabeth. It is not merely by chance that she was hardly ever mentioned in the hundreds of letters he wrote to associates and friends. Since he saw her as his extension, so to speak, he apparently did not consider her life, her personal concerns, or his relationship with her of any real interest, which raises doubts about the degree of intimacy in their relationship. The same pattern of emotional detachment characterized his attitude toward Barbara Bryant, his first significant romantic partner. While she looked up to him as a knowledgeable mentor, ten years her senior, he seemed to be much less involved emotionally. Thus, he did not share with her significant aspects of his life, and when he broke up with her, he did it curtly and abruptly, matter-of-factly explaining that he had things to work out that she could not take part in. And as noted, Kohut's relationships with his closest friends, Palaci, Wadsworth, and McCormick, were likewise characterized by reserve and secretiveness on his part as well as by a lack of reciprocity, where feelings of admiration and/or emotional dependence were unilaterally displayed by his partners to the relationship.

The theme of loneliness and emotional detachment that played such a central role in the life of Kohut underlies three most significant dreams discussed in the case study of Mr. Z. All three are terrifying dreams of emotional distancing and detachment, devoid of any indication of close interpersonal relationships, intimacy, love, or intrapsychic conflict regarding the need for and implications of intimacy and love, although Kohut might not have interpreted the dreams as such.

In one of the dreams, which preceded the second analysis, the image of a meticulously dressed man, holding what looked like an umbrella in one hand and a pair of gloves in the other, appeared against a mountainous landscape. According to Kohut, the dream reflected "the establishment of an idealizing transference" by Mr. Z. (Kohut, 1991/2011, p. 19). However, the lone figure standing isolated, ensconced in his fancy outfit in desolate surroundings, appears to be cold and unapproachable, inaccessible to human interaction, and could thus be seen as reflecting the social isolation and emotional detachment of Mr. Z.

In another dream that Mr. Z. had about his mother, he saw her with her back turned toward him and was horrified at the thought that she was faceless. Kohut interpreted the dream as reflecting the mother's lack of empathy for her son's need for separation and individuation and her "icy withdrawal from him when he attempted to step towards independence" (Kohut, 1991/2011, p. 37). With reference to the dream elsewhere, Kohut (1984) offered a similar interpretation, underscoring his view that it was not the lack of love but rather the lack of empathy that was at issue, where empathy was defined by him as a deep understanding of the other's inner world that did not necessarily involve compassion and concern for or emotional intimacy with the other:

> It is not fear of loss of love that is at stake here. As I explained elsewhere . . . even hatred – that is, human hatred which confirms the victim's humanness – is sustaining. What leads to the human self's destruction, however, is its exposure to the coldness, the indifference of the nonhuman, the nonempathically responding world.
>
> (p. 18)

In a dream about his father, Mr. Z., as a child, saw him, through the slightly open entrance door, returning home after a years-long absence, loaded with gifts for his son. The child, alarmed, closed the door in his face. Kohut linked the dream to the child's deep need for a father figure, unfulfilled all those years, and to the traumatic reunion with the father, "which exposed him suddenly to the potential satisfaction of a central psychological need" (Kohut, 1991/2011, p. 44). The dream reflects the emotional distance between father and son that could not be bridged, notwithstanding the father's wish, as expressed in their reunion, to get closer to his son.

The meaning of separation from a significant figure was likewise interpreted by Kohut in other cases, without due consideration of the aspect of emotional attachment, as illustrated in the analysis of Mr. W. (the psychoanalyst Peter Barglow, presented in the case study as a journalist) (Kohut, 1977). Barglow experienced a traumatic separation from significant attachment figures already in early childhood when, at the age of three and a half, he was actually abandoned by both parents. His father contracted tuberculosis, and his mother chose to stay by the father's bedside and sent little Barglow to his grandparents (disguised in the case study as distant relatives), who lived on a far-off farm. Except for short visits by his mother, Barglow did not see his parents for two and a half years. Kohut reported recurrent regression in the therapeutic process, which occurred whenever a scheduled session was postponed or cancelled for one reason or another. Kohut attributed Barglow's mental difficulties, manifested, inter alia, in irritability, hypochondria, confusion, and dissatisfaction with life, to the failure of his grandparents to show empathy and fulfill his narcissistic needs of mirroring and idealization when taking care of him in his childhood. Barglow himself later said that he felt that his traumatic separation from his parents, which he described as a turning point in his life, was not seen by Kohut as of real importance. The way Kohut saw it, had Barglow's grandparents served as *selfobjects* and met his narcissistic needs, he would have been spared the ensuing mental difficulties, as if emotional attachment to the parents was not of paramount importance in itself and what mattered was merely the functions they were supposed to provide in their interaction with their children.

Kohut similarly played down the importance of emotional attachment to significant attachment figures in his portrayal of Mr. M., an analysand of Anna Ornstein in a case supervised by Kohut (Kohut, 1977). This patient too had a background of traumatic parental abandonment. He was abandoned by his biological mother and at the age of three months was adopted from an orphanage. His adoptive mother fell ill and died when he was 12 years old. After a while, the father married another woman and requested the children not to mention their dead mother. The loss of the adoptive mother or, for that matter, the biological mother, was not seen by Kohut as of critical importance in itself. Instead, he attributed Mr. M.'s mental difficulties to the failure of his adoptive mother to show empathy in his early years and to his adoptive father's failure to provide idealization later on. That is, Kohut did not consider the maternal loss or the ban on processing the loss as decisive factors in the patient's psychological disturbance. As far as he was concerned, significant figures were replaceable, this, as long as their substitutes could provide the subject's narcissistic needs, primarily mirroring and idealization.

The impact of Kohut's schizoidism on his theory

Kohut's theory of self psychology puts the self at the center of psychological existence and thus reflects his narcissistic preoccupation with the self, while the other is not given due consideration. Issues related to the relationship with a separate object, such as the bond of love, the yearning for a close relationship and intimacy with the other, curiosity about the other, envy of the other, rivalry with the other, or loss and grief processes are notably absent from the discussion (Afek, 2019). The concept of *selfobject*, which is fundamental to Kohut's self psychology, calls to mind the notion of the *environment-mother* suggested by Winnicott, the mother whose presence is essential to the development of the self, like oxygen for life, but whose image as a unique and separate human being is considered irrelevant and of no significance in itself. Furthermore, the need for twinship, that is, the need for experiencing similarity to others, is discussed in Kohut's theory in the context of the consolidation of the self and the need for belonging rather than with reference to close relationships between siblings or friends. That is to say, the emphasis is on the function provided by the other, while the relationship with the other, whether emotionally close or distant, is seen as less relevant. Kohut's perception of the other in terms of the function the other serves rather than as a separate and unique human being is reflected, inter alia, in his view of the analyst's role (Magid & Shane, 2017).

The loss of a dearly loved one is an agonizing experience, not least since the departed loved one is irreplaceable. However, Kohut's view of the other as merely serving a function and hence replaceable reflects his failure to acknowledge the significance of a deep and unique relationship with the other. Thus, Kohut (1985) was ambivalent about the concept of "mother" and chose to speak instead of the "empathic responsive matrix" to describe the relationship between a child and a caregiver, "which the child needs for psychological survival and growth" (p. 167). Kohut argued that it did not really matter whether one or several caregivers provided the required empathic environment. To illustrate his argument, Kohut cited a 1951 study by Anna Freud and Sophie Dann on a group of six children who, during their three years in the Terezin concentration camp, were taken care of by successive sets of young women, replaced whenever the former were sent to their death by the Nazis. Playing down the mental impact on the children of the abruptly disappearing, ever-changing mother figures, Kohut suggested that thanks to the empathic responsiveness and devoted care of the young women, the children managed to survive without severe psychotic disorders. Likewise minimizing the significance of close emotional relationships, Kohut (1991/2011) maintained that a mourning process was not to be expected upon the loss of a family member since a familial relationship was a relationship with a *selfobject* rather than with a separate other, and a substitute *selfobject* could be helpful in nourishing and thus restoring the hurt self. To back up his argument, Kohut claimed that Freud himself had acknowledged as much "when he described his own reaction – an absence of mourning – when his grandson died" (p. 310). However, contrary to Kohut's claim, as noted, Freud was devastated by the death of his cherished grandson, so much so that he felt that life had no longer any value for him.

Rothstein (1984/1999, p. 62) critically noted that "Kohut's (1971) emphasis on preoedipal factors and on the formative influence of the parents' personalities results in . . . a somewhat one-sided perspective" that played down the loss of a significant figure, citing Kohut's (1971) own words in this context:

> The absence or loss of the pathological parent may be a wholesome liberation if the child's libidinal resources enable him to move forward and, especially if the other parent, or a parent substitute with a special empathic interest in the threatened child, jumps quickly into the breach and permits a temporary re-establishment of the narcissistic relationship as well as its subsequent gradual dissolution [p. 82].

I quite agree with Rothstein's argument that the loss of a parent is a profoundly traumatic event "with very significant dynamic and structural consequences" (Rothstein, 1984/1999, p. 62) on the child's inner world rather than no more than interference with processes of "transmuting, structure-forming internalization," as argued by Kohut (1971/2009, p. 82) or the loss of an opportunity to facilitate development (Rothstein, 1984/1999, p. 62). Viewing the loss of the other as the loss of part of the self rather than as the loss of a specific significant other, Kohut minimized the significance of the unique relationship maintained with the other. Thus, when analyzing patients who experienced separation or loss, Kohut interpreted their dreams as reflecting their anxiety of disintegration of the self following the separation from a *selfobject* rather than their actual painful experience of separation or loss. By the same token, when discussing the termination of the therapeutic process and relationship later on in his career, Kohut highlighted the "joy" and "liberation of creative energy" upon completion of "a good analysis" rather than the sadness and sorrow over the separation from the analyst (Strozier, 2001, p. 289).

Kohut's view of empathy, a key concept in his theory, seems to be similarly biased. While empathy is generally perceived as related to close interpersonal relationships and associated with a thoughtful and sympathetic attitude toward the other, Kohut saw it as an emotionless diagnostic tool by which the patient's inner world could be observed and understood: "But empathy does not mean love or compassion. Empathy can be used decisively for hateful purposes. I figure out where your weak spots are so I can put the dagger in you" (Kohut, 1985, p. 222). That is, even when discussing the natural human capacity for empathy, Kohut took a defensive position and chose to consider its potentially negative, exploitative, and even malicious aspects.

Kohut's focus on the anxiety of disintegration of the self rather than on anxieties related to relationships with others, for instance, abandonment anxiety, provides further indication of his view of the other as significant only in the context of the function that the other is supposed to serve, namely, the maintenance of the self.

A similarly emotionally distant, narcissistic position was expressed by Kohut when he spontaneously noted in response to a question in an interview, "People ask, 'How should you bring up children?' You can give them a million answers, but the answer really is: 'Be somebody. Then everything will fall in place.'" (Kohut, 1985, p. 243). One may wonder whether by being "somebody" parents can secure the mental health of their children. The answer given by Kohut reflects the importance he attached to achievement, success, and self-realization rather than to warm and loving relationships.

Kohut's difficulty acknowledging the otherness and separateness of the other

There are various indications of Kohut's difficulty acknowledging the otherness and separateness of the other. Thus, he married Elizabeth, who was willing to give up her own identity and, in a sense, served as his extension, devoting herself to taking care of her husband and their son, Thomas, much like Freud's wife Martha. The explanation provided by Kohut for his decision to marry Elizabeth sheds light on the way he saw her, as an inseparable part of himself, fully aligned with him and attuned to his needs. As Kohut wrote in a letter to Aichhorn, "What was for me so decisive was that she knew Vienna, . . . and she knew a little bit what the essential self of mine was" (Strozier, 2001, pp. 100–101). Elizabeth could blend in with the life of Kohut thanks to their shared experiences – her acquaintance with Vienna, her career in a field closely related to psychoanalysis, the fact that she had been a student of Aichhorn, with whom Kohut had undergone analysis and whom he adored – and not least, thanks to her ability to adapt to his needs and live in his shadow as a compliant partner. Kohut's rare references to his wife in his copious correspondence is a further indication of his failure to see her as a separate individual who deserves separate consideration.

Seeking to maintain his sense of dominance as the only or key player, whether in the professional arena or in personal settings, Kohut similarly failed to acknowledge others as separate individuals in their own right. Apparently, it was not by chance that the discussion group that he assembled comprised younger followers who were not likely to challenge his authority and could serve as his subordinate extension. Ina Wolf, one of the group members, pictured Kohut as "a huge arm connected at his fingertips to others with no sense of where his arm ended and the other's began" (Strozier, 2001, p. 276). John Gedo, whom Kohut considered one of the group's luminaries, felt that Kohut expected him to play the role Wilhelm Fliess played for Freud and serve as his *selfobject* and consequently distanced himself from Kohut. As noted, Kohut also took the liberty of interfering with the personal affairs of patients and supervisees, yet again displaying his difficulty acknowledging the otherness and separateness of the other. It seems that his childhood experience with an intrusive mother who ignored his need for separation and individuation was reenacted in his interpersonal relationships later on in life.

Kohut's difficulty acknowledging the otherness and separateness of the other was clearly manifested in his attitude toward other theorists who likewise dealt with the concept of the self, among them, Jung, Carl Rogers, and, in particular, Winnicott, who was a prominent figure in the British Psychoanalytical Society and wrote on the issue about two decades earlier. As critically observed by Philipson (2017), Kohut "presents himself as if he were working in a vacuum, continually breaking new ground" (p. 215). In fact, Kohut himself admitted as much and sought to justify his claim to uniqueness and originality in the preface to *The Restoration of the Self*. Condescendingly dismissing the theorizing of others as nebulous and not well-founded, Kohut (1977) wrote:

> I did not set myself the task of integrating the results of my work with the results of the work of others – results that had been obtained by approaches that are consistent with viewpoints that are different from mine, or that had been formulated within a vague, ambiguous, or shifting theoretical framework.
>
> (p. xxi)

In his last decade, Kohut "stopped reading psychoanalytic literature," and as he told his friend Palaci, he found it "too depressing" to read others' works. "Either you find they say it better or it's not good and you've wasted your time." On another occasion, Kohut explained his decision to refrain from following the writings of other thinkers, noting, "After you turn sixty, . . . you only have time to write and follow your own thoughts and ideas" (Strozier, 2001, p. 243).

Philipson (2017) saw Kohut's rejection of "other theoretical traditions out of hand" as "a defense against vulnerability, a symptom of the grandiose self" (p. 219) and traced his "defensive intellectual isolation" (p. 217) to his Holocaust trauma. Thus, according to Philipson, Kohut's disdainful dismissal of "social psychology" and its focus on external social factors as superficial had to do with his reluctance to acknowledge the impact the traumatizing Holocaust events had on his life. "By asserting his singularity . . . Kohut creates a sense of intellectual invulnerability, and the experience of invulnerability may have had its appeal for someone whose life was forever marked by the Shoah" (p. 216). However, while the Holocaust trauma was no doubt a contributing factor to Kohut's difficulty acknowledging the otherness and separateness of the other, his narcissistic personality was shaped much earlier, in his early childhood and youth, even before the war and his escape from Vienna.

The clinical cases discussed by Kohut provide further evidence of his difficulty acknowledging the otherness and separateness of the other. For the most part, the case studies presented in his writings reflect his own life history, and the analysands are predominantly men, like him (13 men as against 4 women). The mother in the case studies is generally characterized as unstable, unpredictable, evil, and unempathetic, the way Kohut saw his own mother, and hence as the "major pathogenic selfobject" (Strozier, 2001, p. 264). The father is described, just like his own father, as physically absent, emotionally distant, and downtrodden by the mother, yet potentially able to save his son from "the psychological tyranny of the mother" (p. 263), provided he manages to survive the oppressive mother and is given the opportunity to spend more time with his son. While the mother is almost invariably shown in a negative light, the rare moments with the usually absent father are highlighted as formative experiences, with a lasting effect on the patient's personality, apparently due to Kohut's need to idealize his father and picture him as playing a more significant role in his life than he actually did or could do. The portrayal of the father figure by Kohut in a typically positive and even glorifying way is clearly demonstrated in the case of Mr. X. (Kohut, 1977), who was analyzed by a supervisee of Kohut. Like Kohut, Mr. X. grew up with a religious (Christian), overprotective and smothering mother who did not let him break free from her and mirrored his grandiosity only as long as he remained emotionally close to her. At the same time, she prevented him from establishing a meaningful emotional relationship with his father, let alone "relating admiringly to his father" (p. 202). The father, for his part, distanced himself from his son to escape the mother and save himself, but even his limited contact with his son on the few occasions they spent together was described by Kohut as conducive to the mental health of the son. A daydream reported by Mr. X. and the memories it evoked aptly illustrate the point. Driving his car on a trip to the woodlands, Mr. X. got stuck on the way. Realizing that he had run out of gas, he tried to get help, alas, to no avail, and just when he was losing hope, it occurred to him that he had a reserve gasoline can stashed away in the trunk. He filled the tank and drove off, and at that point, woke up from his daydream. He followed the report with an account of his wanderings through the wooded countryside, and pleasant memories of his father were then brought up by association. Mr. X. recalled how his father had taken him for walks in the woods on some of the rare occasions they spent together, reminisced about their shared moments of intimacy, and told the analyst how impressed he was by his father – by his knowledge of the names of trees, his animal tracking skills, and his stories of his hunting prowess as a young man. One may wonder, however, whether those experiences, although so few and rare, could have such a deep impact on the child's psyche and thus save his sanity, as argued by Kohut.

The impact of Kohut's difficulty acknowledging the otherness and separateness of the other on his theory

The key concept, and probably the most innovative concept proposed by Kohut, is the *selfobject*, written as one word, without a hyphen between the words *self* and *object*. It conveys the idea of inseparability of the other and failure to acknowledge the otherness of the other. The other is perceived as an inseparable part or extension of the self, as an arm or leg used in the service of the self, rather than as a separate human being with his own views, needs, thoughts, and emotions. Kohut referred to the *self-selfobject* relationship as oxygen for life, a metaphor first suggested by Balint (1968/2013) to describe the early relationship between infant and mother, whose supportive presence is vital to psychological survival, yet is unnoticed unless unavailable. According to Kohut, *self-selfobject* relationships are maintained from birth to death, shifting throughout life within the *self-selfobject* matrix rather than moving from dependence or symbiosis to independence or autonomy. Kohut saw psychoanalytic theory as biased due to its excessive emphasis, as he perceived it, on the quest for separation from the other. While his contribution to our understanding of *self-selfobject* relationships was highly significant, he failed to address the significance of relationships with a separate other, which are of no less importance in the mental life of the individual. Thus, Kohut maintained that the development of the self was enabled solely by *self-selfobject* relationships while ignoring the key role of relationships with a separate other in the development of the self (Afek, 2019). Indeed, processes of separation and individuation from the parental figure, which involve internalization of the unique characteristics, personality traits, nature, behavior, and attitudes of a primary attachment figure as intrapsychic object representations, are essential to the consolidation of the self. However, Kohut disregarded these processes, and not accidentally. Rather, he envisioned the other as incorporated into and fused with the self, using the foreign protein analogy, whereby ingested beef protein is transmuted in the human body into a digestible form, to describe this transmuting internalization process, as he labeled it. From this perspective, the other's functions are seen as merged into the self, while the other's specific and unique personality characteristics are erased without a trace. Paul Ornstein (1991), Kohut's partner in the development of self psychology, argued that the concept of *object relations* was a misnomer and should be dropped as all relationships were, in fact, *self-selfobject* relationships rather than relationships with a separate object and that the only relevant distinction was between archaic and mature *self-selfobject* relationships. According to Ornstein, this was also applicable to the therapeutic setting and the analyst-patient relationship. Hence, the analyst committed to self psychology should not expect the patient to experience him as a unique and separate individual, but rather serve as the patient's extension or *selfobject*. The analyst's main role was thus seen as being fully attuned to the patient and empathically echoing the patient's emotions and thoughts, in particular, during the typically lengthy 'understanding' stage, while taking care not to express his own feelings, beliefs, or thoughts. This empathic approach to the analytic process reflects the problematic position of self psychology regarding the notion of otherness and separateness as maintained over the decades, even after Kohut's death (Philipson, 2017).

The concept of empathy, central to Kohut's self psychology theory, connotes the ability to put oneself in the other's shoes and understand the other's inner world from his own perspective, which thus provides further indication of the focus of self psychology on the aspect of inseparability in interaction with the other. In the epilogue to the Hebrew translation of Strozier's biography of Kohut (Strozier, 2018), Israeli Kohutian psychoanalyst Raanan Kulka described empathy as a state of consciousness that leads to inseparability between conscious entities. While empathy is no doubt conducive to the therapeutic process, as I discussed at length elsewhere (Afek, 2019) and as critically noted by others (Fosshage, 2003; Goldberg, 1988; Sands, 1997; Shane, 2017; Slavin & Kriegman, 1998; Stern, 2004), Kohut's focus on empathy in psychoanalytic treatment is problematic, specifically as regards the analyst's position vis-à-vis the patient and the analyst's own point of view. Indeed, along with empathic attunement to the patient's subjective experience, it is of the utmost importance that the patient be given the opportunity to cope with otherness, discard his self-centered narcissistic position, and acknowledge otherness as an essential part of mature and reciprocal interpersonal relationships. However, Kohut's self psychology theory considers the encounter with otherness as a threatening experience that should be carefully mediated to the patient rather than as a natural and valuable human experience that contributes to the development of the self – a view that calls to mind Winnicott's perception of otherness and separateness as potentially traumatic for the infant when prematurely experienced.

Furthermore, underlying Kohut's view of the key role of empathy in the therapeutic setting was his belief that psychoanalytic treatment should focus on fulfilling the patient's unfulfilled infantile narcissistic needs. Drawing on his personal experience in early childhood, he developed a theory that matched and answered his own unmet narcissistic needs and proposed an empathic clinical approach attuned to the needs of the patient and designed to provide the patient with grandiosity reinforcing experiences as needed.

Kohut's difficulty acknowledging the otherness and distinctiveness of the other is further reflected in his theory in his disregard of the significance of gender differences for various development processes and in his failure to address the implications of such differences in the context of the child's relationship with the father figure versus his relationship with the mother figure.

Idolized gifted sons, emotionally abandoned – Reflections on the etiology of narcissism

As previously shown, Freud, Winnicott, and Kohut shared prominent narcissistic personality traits, variously displayed by each of them. It would be interesting to explore, based on their early developmental background, whether common contributory factors related to the development of their narcissistic personality traits could be identified. My hypothesis regarding the potential origins of narcissistic personality disorder is presented hereinafter, specifically with reference to the higher levels of personality organization, and is then examined vis-à-vis the life stories of these three pioneers of psychoanalysis, as documented by their biographers and generally known.

In addition to inherent dispositional factors associated with the development of narcissistic personality traits (Ronningstam, 2005), certain early childhood dynamics may raise the risk for the formation of a narcissistic personality at various levels of severity and even lead to the development of narcissistic personality disorder. It is argued that one of the key contributory factors is abrupt and traumatic parental abandonment in early childhood following a blissful spell of a loving relationship with a primary attachment figure in the first year or so of life. The abrupt parental abandonment, followed by chronic emotional abandonment, triggers intense anxiety, and the forsaken infant is left with no way of coping other than defensive self-reliance, which involves perception of the self as omnipotent and invulnerable. Other experiential and environmental factors may come into play in early childhood and further enhance the narcissistic sense of omnipotence and invulnerability, most notably, adoration and idealization of the child on account of an impressive quality, a remarkable talent, an outstanding skill, and the like (for instance, intellectual ingenuity, extraordinary athletic abilities, stunning beauty, or a special role in the parent's life). Often, the adoring and aggrandizing attitude comes in place of love, intimacy, or a real interest in the child's feelings and needs, leaving the child emotionally stranded. Even worse, the adoration and glorification are liable to be accompanied by contradictory messages of deprecation and rejection of other aspects of the child's personality. Such negative messages may be conveyed in various ways – by disregard, contempt, failure to acknowledge the child's feelings of hurt or distress (e.g., telling a child who is sad, 'It's all in your head'), anger, unwillingness to accept a developmental disorder or disability of the child (e.g., learning difficulties and hyperactivity due to attention deficit/hyperactivity disorder [ADHD]), emotional distancing, and so on. The conflicting messages are subsequently reflected, as in a mirror, in the split personality of the narcissist, which is characterized by the presence of two dissociated self-states – the grandiose, omnipotent self and the inferior, vulnerable self (Afek, 2018). The proposed scenario is based on my long clinical experience with narcissistic patients as well as on the theoretical and research literature discussed hereinafter.

Traumatic parental abandonment

A personality split can generally be traced back to an early childhood trauma (Haddock, 2001; McWilliams, 2011; Putnam, 1989). As argued, the narcissistic personality is split into two dissociated self-states, although the narcissist's dissociative experience is not as severe as presented in dissociative identity disorder (Afek, 2018). My view regarding the narcissistic fragmentation of the personality is in line with Bach (1968/1985), Bromberg (2009), Cooper (1998), Goldberg (1999), Horowitz (2013), Miller (1981), and Symington (1993). Orange (2011) referred at length to Ferenczi's discussion of "the narcissistic dissociation of the self" (citing Ferenczi, 1931 and Ferenczi, 1949), which he ascribed to traumatic sexual abuse in early childhood. In this context, Orange quoted Ferenczi's account of a typical dream quite often reported by his patients, the dream of the clever baby. According to Ferenczi, the dream, concerning a highly capable precocious infant or young child, reflected a narcissistic self-splitting defensively used by the traumatized child, where one part of the self remained vulnerable and immature while the other part developed a precocious maturity and assumed the role of a parentified child, displaying an adult-like emotional intelligence. Orange noted the similarity between Ferenczi's "clever baby" and Alice Miller's "gifted child," who, as the narcissistic survivors of early trauma emotionally familiar with the omnipotent position of the caretaking child, were likely to find their calling in the therapeutic professions.

Unlike Ferenczi, who focused on sexual abuse as the key factor at the root of narcissistic dissociation of the self, I believe that the trauma related to narcissistic dissociation is of a different nature and has to do primarily with parental abandonment in early childhood, in most cases, abrupt abandonment that is followed by chronic emotional abandonment. In fact, research shows that traumatic sexual abuse in early childhood is one of the main factors relevant to the etiology of borderline personality disorder (Bradley et al., 2005), while it is not necessarily related to the development of narcissistic personality disorder. Furthermore, it was shown that people who grew up in dysfunctional and chaotic families with unstable and neglecting parents were at a higher risk of borderline personality disorder (Widom et al., 2009). On the other hand, in many cases, people with a narcissistic personality were brought up in more stable and functional families (Glickauf-Hughes, 1997).

Symington (1993) highlighted trauma as a major cause of narcissism. According to Symington, early childhood trauma leads the traumatized infant to turn away from the *lifegiver,* that is, the parental figure, and deny his emotional need for the *lifegiver*. While Symington did not explicitly point to traumatic parental abandonment as a prime cause of narcissism, his discussion of the nature of trauma and the few illustrative examples presented in that context indicate that he saw parental abandonment, whether actual or emotional, as one of the main contributory factors. Inter alia, Symington wrote:

> A man of 50 might be prepared for the death of his mother; a one-year-old child is not. There is a preparation through life for particular losses, separations, deaths, and so on. The essence of trauma is that a stability based on steady expectation has been shattered.
>
> (p. 74)

Yet the infant's rejection of the *lifegiver* and denial of his emotional need for the *lifegiver* can only be understood in the context of a traumatic emotional abandonment by the parental figure, who proves to be unreliable and unworthy of trust. The infant thus has no choice but to rely on himself at that early and critical stage in life and hold on to illusory thoughts of grandiosity, as far as such thoughts can be entertained at that early developmental stage. Rothstein (1984/1999) discussed parental abandonment as a potential cause of narcissism, although not necessarily the single or major cause. Rothstein argued that apart from parental emotional abandonment, actual parental loss in early childhood was often at the root of adult narcissism, and since at that early stage the child lacked the emotional and cognitive resources for coping with the trauma, he could hardly recover from the loss. Similarly, Kealy and Ogrodniczuk (2014) cited parental abandonment in early childhood as a possible contributory factor, noting that mentalization deficits typical of the narcissistic personality reflected an early traumatic experience of parental abandonment. Hagman (2016), who dealt at length with the issue of bereavement and mourning, noted the link between the difficulty acknowledging the otherness of the other – one of the three core features of the narcissistic personality previously discussed (and addressed in more detail in Chapter 3) – and parental abandonment or loss in early childhood. While Hagman did not explicitly characterize his patients as narcissists, their portrayal is consistent with the characterization of the narcissistic personality. They were described by Hagman as oblivious of the analyst's presence in the therapeutic setting, as if they were alone in the room or as if a glass partition separated them from the analyst, who was given the feeling of being an insubstantial shadow or a ghost.

As noted, I believe that narcissism has its origins in traumatic parental abandonment in early childhood that occurs following an initial phase of a close emotional relationship between the infant and a primary attachment figure. In fact, the grandiose, omnipotent sense of self underlying the narcissistic personality cannot possibly develop in the absence of such an intimate relationship, where the primary attachment figure, usually the mother, is fully attuned to the needs of the infant. This argument is consistent with Winnicott's view of the beneficial role of the *good enough mother* as essential to the development and consolidation of the grandiose self in the early months of life. Furthermore, the impressive ego forces and highly developed defense mechanisms displayed by many of the narcissists (Blatt, 2008), their remarkable achievements, high motivation, courage, creativity, and leadership capacity (Maccoby, 2004) indicate that those narcissists with a higher level of personality organization experienced a primary stage of a close emotional relationship with a loving and caring primary attachment figure who gratified their deepest needs. One may wonder, then, how parental abandonment fits in this picture of healthy parent-child relationships. The reasons for parental abandonment following such a happy period of emotional attachment are varied. It could be the narcissistic personality of the parental figure who finds it difficult to accept the child's quest for independence and separation and reacts by emotional distancing. It could also be external circumstances such as illness, divorce, economic difficulties, or the loss of a sibling that abruptly put an end to the blissful parent-child relationship and subsequently expose the child to chronic emotional abandonment.

Conflicting messages

The experience of grandiosity and omnipotence is contingent on constant narcissistic supply, which is essential to sustaining and reinforcing the grandiose sense of self. It is not surprising, then, that narcissists are often endowed with an attractive quality, a remarkable skill, or a unique talent by virtue of which they gain the admiration of others (Diamond et al., 2022). As children, they are adored and adulated by their parents for their good looks, athletic achievements, cleverness, and so on, and at times, it is the place or role of the child in the family rather than a striking trait that earns him a privileged status, as my clinical experience shows. Thus, an only child enjoys the parents' exclusive attention and affection, not having to share it with siblings; a girl born after several boys is cherished as the little princess; and a parentified child is instilled with an omnipotent sense of self (Ronningstam, 2005). However, quite often, the privileged status comes with a heavy price. As observed by Orange (2011, citing Ferenczi) as well as by Miller (1981), the highly capable parentified child or uniquely gifted child is required to display precocious maturity, give up his own needs, and act as a little adult or a young carer. Mitchell (1986) highlighted the aggrandizing parental messages, conveyed regardless of their underlying illusory nature and the child's emotional immaturity, as a key factor in the formation of the narcissistic personality. A child exposed to parental illusory overvaluation as a dominant feature of his relationship with the parent is liable to adopt a narcissistic mode of relatedness as an adult and find it difficult to maintain interpersonal relationships that do not revolve around his sense of grandiosity and omnipotence.

The inflated sense of self typical of the narcissist may, at times, be traced back to the high status (economic, social, professional, etc.) of his family rather than to a special personal trait or quality, as I have found in my clinical work with narcissistic patients. In this case, narcissistic personality traits may be displayed by patients' siblings as well, while the severity of narcissistic pathology is dependent on other contributory factors, first and foremost, as argued, parental emotional abandonment.

The omnipotent narcissistic experience, which originates in traumatic abandonment in early childhood, is then enhanced by constant idealization and aggrandizement throughout childhood. Otway and Vignoles (2006) noted an apparent inconsistency between different psychotherapeutic theories regarding the etiology of adult narcissism – those that trace narcissistic pathology to excessive parental adoration and adulation or overindulgence of the child, who is seen as superior to others and thus entitled to a privileged status (for instance, Brummelman et al., 2015; Millon & Everly, 1985) and those that cite the emotional detachment of the parental figure or a traumatic experience involving the parental figure in early childhood as the key factors at the root of narcissistic personality disorder (for instance, Kernberg, 1975; Symington, 1993). Otway and Vignoles (2006) studied the issue based on the childhood recollections of 120 adult respondents. They found that parental idealization and aggrandizement as well as parental coldness, detachment, and devaluation, often simultaneously present, were predictors of adult narcissism. Their findings support my argument regarding the effect of conflicting parental messages on the development of narcissism. As my clinical experience shows, such conflicting messages, which trigger narcissistic dissociation and self-splitting, are variously conveyed. Thus, parents may admire and adulate certain traits of a child while displaying a critical and negative attitude about his personality, needs, or behavior. In other instances, one of the parents may be on the admiring and adulating side while the other parent is on the censorious, devaluing side (Behary & Dieckmann, 2013). And at times, the parents may idealize and aggrandize their child while the environment conveys belittling and devaluing messages for various reasons, for instance, when the child's family belongs to a socially marginalized group (e.g., an ethnic minority) or is of a low socioeconomic status, or when the child has a physical disability, and so on. Paulina Kernberg (1998) identified certain risk factors for the development of narcissistic pathology, noting, inter alia, the conflicting messages that adopted children are exposed to – while cherished by their adoptive parents, they are scarred by their abandonment by their biological parents.

In conclusion, a combination of factors, simultaneously present, contribute to the development of narcissistic pathology, and the further these factors come into play, the more severe the narcissistic pathology. Parental abandonment in infancy occurring after a close relationship with a parental figure has been experienced leads to desperate recourse to defensive self-reliance. The associated grandiose sense of self is nourished and enhanced by adoration and idealization of the child, while simultaneous rejection, deprecation, or emotional detachment give rise to a vulnerable, inferior, and flawed experience of the self, resulting in an unrealistic self-perception. The constant shift between these conflicting experiences is subsequently reflected in the sharp fluctuations in the narcissist's sense of self in reaction to any real or imagined success or failure.

The origins of Freud's, Winnicott's, and Kohut's narcissism

Freud

Traumatic parental abandonment

As the firstborn child and son, Freud enjoyed affectionate and adoring motherly attention in the first year and a half of his life. However, all that came to an end when his baby brother, Julius, died several months after birth, leaving his mother in profound grief and thus emotionally unavailable at a critical stage of his development. The successive births soon afterward of his siblings, Anna and four other sisters and his youngest brother, Alexander, inevitably taxed his mother's time and energy and diverted her attention from little Freud. Furthermore, his abrupt separation from his nanny, to whom he was deeply attached, when he was just two and a half years old, at about the time his sister Anna was born, intensified his experience of emotional abandonment. Atwood and Stolorow (1993) noted the far-reaching impact of the emotional abandonment experienced by Freud so early in life, which was in striking contrast to his primary experience of loving motherly care and thus explained his ambivalent feelings about his mother and difficulty acknowledging his negative feelings toward her, lest he would be abandoned once again. In this context, the authors cited one of his childhood dreams, reported in Freud's (1913) *The Interpretation of Dreams*. In the dream, Freud saw his mother carried by people with birds' beaks and laid dead on a bed, and at that point, he woke up in horror. While Freud interpreted the dream as reflecting his concealed sexual wishes about his mother, Atwood and Stolorow observed, and rightly so, that based on Freud's own theorizing on dreams of death, the dream could be interpreted as expressing his deep-seated, unacknowledged hostility and aggression toward his mother and, in fact, a death wish against her. Be that as it may, in my view, the dream reflects Freud's feelings of anxiety and agony related to his traumatic abandonment in infancy by the mother figure (his mother as well as his nanny) – a traumatic experience from which he never recovered.

The myth of Oedipus, with whom Freud deeply identified, could shed more light on his traumatic experience of parental abandonment. While Freud consciously identified with the phallic masculinity represented by Oedipus, the valiant male warrior, the story of Oedipus, the ill-fated baby doomed to fulfill a prophecy that he would kill his father and marry his mother and consequently abandoned to his death by his parents, apparently resonated with Freud's own experience of early childhood abandonment and thus prompted his unconscious identification with Oedipus the forsaken baby.

It is noteworthy that while Freud deeply mourned his father's death, he felt a certain measure of relief upon the death of his mother and was not even present at her funeral. Was it because of his negative feelings toward her over his emotional abandonment by her, or did he find it too difficult to deal once again with the experience of maternal abandonment, that time, ultimate abandonment? On various occasions, Freud referred to his fear that he would die before his mother, Was it due to projective identification that he felt that he could not possibly abandon her as her pain would be unbearable, as intense as the pain he felt when emotionally abandoned in infancy? There are no clear-cut answers to these questions, but as acknowledged by Freud himself, his reaction to his mother's death was unusual and unnatural.

Conflicting messages

There is ample evidence of the adoration and adulation of Freud and of his preferential status in the family as a child prodigy and as the eldest and, for several years, the only son. He was the favorite child of his mother, *mein goldener Sigi*, as she called him (Atwood & Stolorow, 1993, p. 38, citing Jones, 1953). Yet it seems that Freud's mother was a self-centered, narcissistic, and domineering woman who used little Freud as her extension for her own self-aggrandizement (Rubin, 1998). It is thus in doubt to what extent she was attentive and responsive to his emotional needs. Her emotional detachment following the death of her second son, Julius, in infancy (and loss of her brother around that time) coupled with her frequent pregnancies, which deprived Freud of her exclusive attention, were most probably perceived by Freud as reflecting rejection on the part of his mother.

At the same time, Freud's father appears to have been a less dominant figure in his life, due to both his mild, docile temper and limited involvement in child rearing (common among fathers at the time). To the extent that he was mentioned by Freud, it was mostly in the context of incidents of disapproval and deprecation that left an indelible mark on Freud's soul. Freud's recurring dream of a humiliating childhood incident described earlier, where he urinated in the presence of his parents and was harshly rebuked by his father, indicates that such situations were variously experienced by Freud throughout his childhood. Indeed, it apparently revealed just the tip of the iceberg of Freud's troubled relationship with his father, who not only repeatedly belittled his son but, being perceived by Freud as weak and passive, failed to present a father figure for identification and thus undermined Freud's sense of self-worth and competence (sending Freud to look elsewhere for valiant heroes like Hannibal to identify with).

Along with the conflicting parental messages, Freud was exposed to the virulent anti-Semitism of the era, which denigrated Jews as flawed and inferior, and internalized the demeaning anti-Semitic stereotypes (Aron & Starr, 2013; Boyarin et al., 2003). Thus, when he reached the age of 16, Freud decided to change his original Jewish name, Sigismund Schlomo – "Sigismund was an unfortunate choice, a comic name popular in German-language jokes about Jews" – and "amended Sigismund to the more dignified Sigmund" (Ferris, 1997, p. 15).

Winnicott

Traumatic parental abandonment

Winnicott's first years of life are shrouded in fog, this, not least due to the near-idyllic, albeit not necessarily true-to-reality picture of his childhood that Winnicott and his second wife Clare painted. While there is no evidence of actual parental abandonment or of external circumstances that could lead to abrupt and traumatic parental abandonment during Winnicott's formative years, there are indications that Winnicott grew up with a depressive mother, as implied, inter alia, by Winnicott himself in his poem *The Tree* (Phillips, 1988/2007; Rodman, 2003). It may thus be assumed that Winnicott's mother was emotionally detached and unavailable when he needed her most, in his infancy and childhood. Another indication of the emotional withdrawal of Winnicott's mother already early on was provided by Marion Milner (as cited by Rodman, 2003). Commenting on a well-known drawing by Winnicott of a mother and her infant, where the mother's backbone is plainly depicted, Milner wondered whether it represented "his mother's father's 'forbidding penis' which stood between herself and Donald, that is, if it was a stricture originating in the attitude of her father that had led to a conflict when she found herself stimulated by her son's feeding" and thus weaned him at a rather early stage, as Winnicott once told Milner (p. 14). However, as noted, it could be as well the emotional state of Winnicott's depressive mother rather than a mental conflict over moral strictures that accounted for her detachment. Further indication of the emotional distance between Winnicott and his mother (and sisters) was suggested by Clare (Winnicott, 1989/2018):

> Because Donald was so very much the youngest member of the Winnicott household (even the youngest boy cousin living opposite was older than he) and because he was so much loved and was in himself lovable, it seems likely that a deliberate effort was made, particularly on the part of his mother and sisters, not to spoil him. While this did not deprive him of feeling loved, it did I think deprive him of some intimacy and closeness that he needed.
>
> (pp. 6–7)

It appears that Winnicott's father, a domineering and demanding person with narcissistic characteristics, who was preoccupied with his business affairs and numerous public duties, was not emotionally available either. As noted, Winnicott felt let down and abandoned by his father, who left him to the care of the women surrounding him – his mother, two elder sisters, an aunt, a nanny, and a governess (Phillips, 1988/2007). The absence of a father figure during Winnicott's early years is clearly reflected in his theory of the parent-infant relationship, which revolves around the *good enough mother* and her vital role in early development while virtually ignoring the role of the father figure in the emotional development of the infant.

Conflicting messages

As the youngest child and only son in the family, born several years after two sisters, Winnicott enjoyed a special status at home, enhanced by virtue of his endearing, loveable personality. Furthermore, Winnicott saw himself as the savior of his depressive mother, tasked with the role of enlivening her and curing "her inward death," as he wrote in his poem *The Tree* (Phillips, 1988/2007; Rodman, 2003) – a role that strengthened his grandiose, omnipotent sense of self.

At the same time, faced with the depression and emotional withdrawal of his mother, Winnicott most probably felt rejected by her and unworthy of her love. He apparently felt rejected by his father as well. While Winnicott described his father in a positive light, his father's emotional detachment and negative, belittling attitude emerge between the lines, as reflected in a childhood memory related by Winnicott. It appears that his father used to tease him over a wax doll called Rosie that belonged to his sisters, parodying a popular song (Phillips, 1988/2007, p. 27):

> *Rosie said to Donald*
> *I love you*
> *Donald said to Rosie*
> *I don't believe you do.*

Winnicott recalled that irritated and humiliated, he smashed the doll's nose with a croquet mallet. His vivid memory of the episode, which had to do with a feminine object (the doll) and a vulnerable emotion (love) and provoked his enraged reaction, points to the underlying derogatory message regarding his femininity and failure to live up to his father's expectations. Similar critical messages about Winnicott's deficient masculinity, apparently conveyed by the environment, could explain his need to shake off his image as "too nice" at the age of nine and adopt a seemingly masculine, aggressive manner.

Kohut

Traumatic parental abandonment

Kohut's early months of life, until he was a little over a year, were probably his best and happiest. As the first and only son, he enjoyed the full attention and affection of both his parents. His father, a warm person with a positive mindset, had a close and meaningful relationship with his little son. In those early days, Kohut experienced a good and healthy relationship with his mother as well. As noted by Strozier (2001), citing Kohut's (1991/2011) self-description in the autobiographical case of Mr. Z., however "severely distorted" her personality turned out to be later on,

> she was young and full of vitality when Heinz was born. She had an "intense relationship" with her little boy. As long as he remained a baby, the "interweaving of her with him" seemed to bring out her "healthiest attitudes." He was the "apple of her eye."
>
> (Strozier, 2001, p. 12)

However, following the enlistment of Kohut's father at the outbreak of World War I, the blissful family life "came crashing down before Heinz could even talk. It was truly a paradise lost" (p. 13). The abrupt separation and four-year absence of the father, except for short visits during the war years, must have been traumatic for little Heinz, all the more so considering the significant role his father played in his first year of life. The events exacted a heavy toll on Kohut's mother, who was unexpectedly left alone with a one-year-old baby, cut off from her beloved husband. Never recovering, she became emotionally detached and unavailable. While she took care of the day-to-day needs of her son (indeed, to the point of being overly intrusive, as previously described) and saw to his education, her emotional absence in a critical stage of his development and failure to respond to his emotional needs compounded his early childhood abandonment trauma. As noted, she failed to show empathy for his need for separation and individuation and reacted by "icy withdrawal" whenever he tried to move toward independence. A shocking account of her alienation was provided in the horrific dream of the faceless mother reported by Mr. Z. (Kohut, 1991/2011). She likewise ignored his need for socializing with peers (as noted, she did not send him to school until the fifth grade and kept him socially isolated in the following years as well). The reunion with his father after the war could not compensate for the years of absence. Weighed down by the war horrors, his father lost his once lively vitality. Dejected, reserved, and emotionally unavailable, he left Kohut alone with his emotionally detached, unstable, mentally disturbed mother. Kohut thus experienced chronic emotional abandonment throughout his childhood and youth, with no corrective experience and no healing for the abrupt parental abandonment in infancy.

Conflicting messages

As an only child and only son, Kohut was adored and adulated by his parents and given the feeling that he was special and cherished. Once he remained alone with his mother after the enlistment of his father, little Heinz became the focus of her life. Indeed, he served as an inseparable extension, as it were, of his mother, sleeping next to her at night and spending most of the day with her at home, with virtually no visits from friends, his or hers. His isolation from the external world by his mother could be attributed to her paranoid personality, manifested as full-blown paranoid psychosis in her last years of life. Kohut thus found himself in the role of a substitute for his missing father in the relationship with his mother – an experience that most probably fostered his inflated sense of self-worth.

However, along with the aggrandizing messages, the paternal abandonment in infancy followed by the maternal emotional detachment and hostile withdrawal in reaction to any manifestation of individuality and independence on the part of Kohut left him feeling rejected and unwanted. His experience of rejection was further intensified by his forced social isolation and associated feelings of loneliness and exclusion. An indication of his negative self-image in childhood and, in fact, doubts about his own sanity may be found in his feelings of relief and liberation, of which he spoke frequently, upon the confirmation of his mother's psychotic paranoia. It was important to him to have it confirmed that she – not he – was the "crazy" one. His negative self-experience persisted even after his father's return from the war. As noted, his father, traumatized by the war horrors and emotionally withdrawn, could not possibly contribute to enhancing his self-image.

What is more, like Freud, Kohut was exposed to the rife anti-Semitism of the time and internalized its deprecating messages, which further hurt his sense of self and, later on, led to his denial of his Jewish origins.

Note

1 As noted elsewhere in this book (citing Kohut, 1984, and Togashi & Kottler, 2021), a slight change of focus can be discerned in Kohut's later writings, where rather than emphasizing the role of twinship in sustaining a cohesive self, Kohut referred to its relational aspect, redefining twinship as the need to be human "among other human beings."

References

Afek, O. (2018). The split narcissist: The grandiose self versus the inferior self. *Psychoanalytic Psychology, 35*(2), 231–236. https://doi.org/10.1037/pap0000161

Afek, O. (2019). Reflections on Kohut's theory of self psychology and pathological narcissism – Limitations and concerns. *Psychoanalytic Psychology, 36*(2), 166–172. https://doi.org/10.1037/pap0000201

Aron, L. (1996). *A meeting of minds: Mutuality in psychoanalysis*. The Analytic Press. https://read.amazon.com/?asin=B0B9KHXHZ1&ref_=kwl_kr_iv_rec_1

Aron, L., & Starr, K. (2013). *A psychotherapy for the people: Toward a progressive psychoanalysis*. Routledge/Taylor & Francis Group.

Atwood, G. E., & Stolorow, R. D. (1993). *Faces in a cloud: Intersubjectivity in personality theory*. Jason Aronson.

Bach, S. (1985). *Narcissistic states and the therapeutic process*. Jason Aronson.

Balint, M. (2013). *The basic fault: Therapeutic aspects of regression*. Routledge. (Original work published 1968)

Behary, W., & Dieckmann, E. (2013). Schema therapy for pathological narcissism. In J. S. Ogrodniczuk (Ed.), *Understanding and treating pathological narcissism*. American Psychological Association.

Benjamin, J. (1999). Recognition and destruction: An outline of intersubjectivity. In S. A. Mitchell & L. Aron (Eds.), *Relational psychoanalysis: The emergence of a tradition* (pp. 181–210). Routledge.
Blatt, S. J. (2008). *Polarities of experience: Relatedness and self-definition in personality development, psychopathology, and the therapeutic process*. American Psychological Association.
Boyarin, D., Itzkovitz, D., & Pellegrini, A. (Eds.). (2003). *Queer theory and the Jewish question*. Columbia University Press.
Bradley, R., Jenei, J., & Westen, D. (2005). Etiology of borderline personality disorder: Disentangling the contributions of intercorrelated antecedents. *Journal of Nervous and Mental Disease, 193*(1), 24–31. https://doi.org/10.1097/01.nmd.0000149215.88020.7c
Breuer, J., & Freud, S. (1995). *Studies on hysteria* (J. Strachey, Ed. & Trans., in collaboration with Anna Freud, Standard Edition, Vol. 2, pp. 1–335). Hogarth Press. (Original work published 1895)
Bromberg, P. M. (2009). Discussion of Robert Grossmark's case of Pamela. *Psychoanalytic Dialogues, 19*(1), 31–38.
Brummelman, E., Thomaes, S., Nelemans, S. A., Orobio de Castro, B., Overbeek, G., & Bushman, B. J. (2015). Origins of narcissism in children. *Proceedings of the National Academy of Sciences, 112*(12), 3659–3662.
Cooper, A. (1998). Further developments in the clinical diagnosis of narcissistic personality disorder. In E. Ronningstam (Ed.), *Disorders of narcissism: Diagnostic, clinical, and empirical implications* (pp. 53–74). American Psychiatric Press.
Diamond, D., Yeomans, F. E., Stern, B. L., & Kernberg, O. F. (2022). *Treating pathological narcissism with transference-focused psychotherapy*. The Guilford Press.
Edmundson, M. (2007). *The death of Sigmund Freud: The legacy of his last days*. Bloomsbury.
Ferenczi, S., & Dupont, J. (Ed.). (1988). *The clinical diary of Sándor Ferenczi* (M. Balint & N. Z. Jackson, Trans.). Harvard University Press.
Ferris, P. (1997). *Dr Freud: A life*. Random House.
Fosshage, J. L. (2003). Contextualizing self psychology and relational psychoanalysis: Bi-directional influence and proposed syntheses. *Contemporary Psychoanalysis, 39*(3), 411–448. https://doi.org/10.1080/00107530.2003.10747214
Freud, S. (1913). *The interpretation of dreams* (A. A. Brill, Trans.). The Macmillan Company. https://doi.org/10.1037/10561-000
Freud, S. (1917). *Mourning and Melancholia* (J. Strachey, Ed. & Trans., in collaboration with Anna Freud, Standard Edition, Vol. 14, pp. 243–258). The Hogarth Press and the Institute of Psychoanalysis.
Freud, S. (1920). *A general introduction to psychoanalysis* (G. S. Hall, Trans.). Horace Liveright.
Freud, S. (1921). *Group psychology and the analysis of the ego* (J. Strachey, Ed. & Trans., Standard Edition, Vol. 18, pp. 65–144). The International Psychoanalytical Library.
Freud, S. (1923). *The ego and the id and other works* (J. Strachey, Trans., Standard Edition, Vol. 19). The Hogarth Press and the Institute of Psychoanalysis.
Freud, S. (1926). *The question of lay analysis* (J. Strachey, Trans., Standard Edition, Vol. 20, pp. 177–258). The Hogarth Press and the Institute of Psychoanalysis.
Freud, S. (1955). *The Moses of Michelangelo* (J. Strachey, Ed., & Trans., in collaboration with Anna Freud, Standard Edition, Vol. 13, pp. 211–238). The Hogarth Press and the Institute of Psychoanalysis. (Original work published 1914)
Freud, S. (1992). *Letters of Sigmund Freud* (E. L. Freud, Ed.; T. Stern & J. Stern, Trans.). Dover Publications. (Original work published 1960)
Gay, P. (1998). *Freud: A life for our time*. W.W. Norton & Company. https://read.amazon.com/?asin=B007NNSU36&ref_=kwl_kr_iv_rec_14

Glickauf-Hughes, C. (1997). Etiology of the masochistic and narcissistic personality. *American Journal of Psychoanalysis, 57*(2), 141–148. https://doi.org/10.1023/a:1024796310426
Goldberg, A. I. (1988). *A fresh look at psychoanalysis: The view from self psychology* (1st ed.). Routledge. https://doi.org/10.4324/9780203766378
Goldberg, A. I. (1999). *Being of two minds: The vertical split in psychoanalysis and psychotherapy*. The Analytic Press. https://read.amazon.com/?asin=B00DL1U6GI&ref_=kwl_kr_iv_rec_1
Goldman, D. (1993). *In search of the real: The origins and originality of D. W. Winnicott*. Jason Aronson.
Guntrip, H. (1992). *Schizoid phenomena, object relations and the self*. Karnac Books. https://read.amazon.com/?asin=B005RX17FW&ref_=kwl_kr_iv_rec_15 (Original work published 1968)
Haddock, D. (2001). *The dissociative identity disorder sourcebook*. McGraw Hill Professional.
Hagman, G. (Ed.). (2016). *New models of bereavement theory and treatment: New mourning*. Routledge/Taylor & Francis Group.
Hopkins, L. B. (1998). D. W. Winnicott's analysis of Masud Khan: A preliminary study of failures of object usage. *Contemporary Psychoanalysis, 34*(1), 5–47.
Hopkins, L. B. (2004). Red shoes, untapped madness, and Winnicott on the cross: An interview with Marion Milner. *Annual of Psychoanalysis, 32*, 233–243.
Horowitz, M. (2013). Prototypical formulation of pathological narcissism. In J. S. Ogrodniczuk (Ed.), *Understanding and treating pathological narcissism*. American Psychological Association. https://read.amazon.com/?asin=B00B1W2FAO&ref_=kwl_kr_iv_rec_1
Issroff, J. (2018). *Donald Winnicott and John Bowlby: Personal and professional perspectives* (with contributions from B. Hauptmann & C. Reeves). Routledge. (Original work published 2005)
Jung, C. G. (1989). *Memories, dreams, reflections* (A. Jaffé, Ed.; R. Winston & C. Winston, Trans.; rev. ed.). Vintage Books. https://read.amazon.com/?asin=B004FYZK52&ref_=kwl_kr_iv_rec_2 (Original work published 1961)
Kahr, B., & Bechdel, A. (2016). *Tea with Winnicott*. Routledge.
Kealy, D., & Ogrodniczuk, J. S. (2014). Pathological narcissism and the obstruction of love. *Psychodynamic Psychiatry, 42*(1), 101–119. https://doi.org/10.1521/pdps.2014.42.1.101
Kernberg, O. F. (1975). *Borderline conditions and pathological narcissism*. Rowman & Littlefield. https://read.amazon.com/?asin=B00BZAMWA0&ref_=kwl_kr_iv_rec_23
Kernberg, P. F. (1998). Developmental aspects of normal and pathological narcissism. In E. F. Ronningstam (Ed.), *Disorders of narcissism: Diagnostic, clinical, and empirical implications* (pp. 103–120). American Psychiatric Association.
Kohut, H. (1966). Forms and transformations of narcissism. *Journal of the American Psychoanalytic Association, 14*(2), 243–272.
Kohut, H. (1977). *The restoration of the self*. International Universities Press.
Kohut, H. (1984). *How does analysis cure?* (A. Goldberg, Ed., with P. E. Stepansky). The University of Chicago Press. https://read.amazon.com/?asin=B015KJZF8M&ref_=kwl_kr_iv_rec_1
Kohut, H. (1985). *Self psychology and the humanities: Reflections on a new psychoanalytic approach* (C. B. Strozier, Ed.). Norton.
Kohut, H. (2009). *The analysis of the self: A systematic approach to the psychoanalytic treatment of narcissistic personality disorders*. The University of Chicago Press. https://read.amazon.com/?asin=B00FXMPJKG&ref_=kwl_kr_iv_rec_3 (Original work published 1971)
Kohut, H. (2011). *The search for the self: Selected writings of Heinz Kohut: 1978–1981. Vol. 4* (P. H. Ornstein, Ed.). Karnac Books. https://read.amazon.com/?asin=B00582LHI4&ref_=kwl_kr_iv_rec_5 (Original work published 1991)

Little, M. I. (1990). *Psychotic anxieties and containment: A personal record of an analysis with Winnicott*. Jason Aronson.

Maccoby, M. (2004). Narcissistic leaders: The incredible pros, the inevitable cons. In A. Hooper (Ed.), *Leadership perspectives* (pp. 31–39). Routledge.

Magid, B., & Shane, E. (2017). Relational self psychology. *Psychoanalysis, Self and Context, 12*(1), 3–19.

Masson, J. M. (2012). *Against therapy: Emotional tyranny and the myth of psychological healing*. Untreed Reads Publishing. https://read.amazon.com/?asin=B008KPZRDW&ref_=kwl_kr_iv_rec_17 (Original work published 1988)

McWilliams, N. (2006). Some thoughts about schizoid dynamics. *Psychoanalytic Review, 93*(1), 1–24.

McWilliams, N. (2011). *Psychoanalytic diagnosis: Understanding personality structure in the clinical process* (2nd ed.). Guilford Press.

Miller, A. (1981). *The drama of the gifted child: The search for the true self* (R. Ward, Trans.). Basic Books.

Millon, T., & Everly, G. S. (1985). *Personality and its disorders: A biosocial learning approach*. John Wiley & Sons.

Mitchell, S. A. (1986). The wings of Icarus: Illusion and the problem of narcissism. *Contemporary Psychoanalysis, 22*(1), 107–132.

Mitchell, S. A. (1993). *Hope and dread in psychoanalysis*. Basic Books.

Mitchell, S. A. (2023). *Relationality: From attachment to intersubjectivity*. Routledge. https://read.amazon.com/?asin=B0B92S5PVW&ref_=kwl_kr_iv_rec_3 (Original work published 2000)

Mitchell, S.A., & Black, M.J. (2016). *Freud and beyond: A history of modern psychoanalytic thought*. Basic Books. https://read.amazon.com/?asin=B06XBVPQGS&ref_=kwl_kr_iv_rec_1 (Original work published 1995)

Modell, A. H. (1975). A narcissistic defence against affects and the illusion of self-sufficiency. *The International Journal of Psychoanalysis, 56*, 275–282.

Ogden, T. H. (1990). *The matrix of the mind: Object relations and the psychoanalytic dialogue*. Karnac Books. https://read.amazon.com/?asin=B005RX128O&ref_=kwl_kr_iv_rec_34 (Original work published 1986)

Orange, D. M. (2011). *The suffering stranger: Hermeneutics for everyday clinical practice*. Routledge.

Ornstein, P. H. (1991). Why self psychology is not an object relations theory: Clinical and theoretical considerations. In A. Goldberg (Ed.), *The evolution of self psychology: Progress in self psychology* (Vol. 7, pp. 17–29). The Analytic Press.

Otway, L. J., & Vignoles, V. L. (2006). Narcissism and childhood recollections: A quantitative test of psychoanalytic predictions. *Personality and Social Psychology Bulletin, 32*(1), 104–116.

Philipson, I. (2017). Fearing the theoretical other: The legacy of Kohut's erasure of the analyst's trauma. *Psychoanalysis, Self and Context, 12*(3), 211–220.

Phillips, A. (2007). *Winnicott*. Penguin Books. https://read.amazon.com/?asin=B002RI99FA&ref_=kwl_kr_iv_rec_1 (Original work published 1988)

Putnam, F. W. (1989). *Diagnosis and treatment of multiple personality disorder*. Guilford Press.

Reeves, C. (2004). On being "intrinsical": A Winnicott enigma. *American Imago, 61*(4), 427–455.

Renik, O. (2006). *Practical psychoanalysis for therapists and patients*. Other Press. https://read.amazon.com/?asin=B003WUYOZC&ref_=kwl_kr_iv_rec_1

Rodman, F. R. (2003). *Winnicott: Life and work*. Perseus Publishing.

Rolnik, E. (2019). *Sigmund Freud – Letters*. Modan. [Hebrew]

Ronningstam, E. (2005). *Identifying and understanding the narcissistic personality*. Oxford University Press.

Rosenfeld, H. (1964). On the psychopathology of narcissism: A clinical approach. *The International Journal of Psychoanalysis, 45*, 332–337.

Rothstein, A. (1999). *The narcissistic pursuit of perfection* (2nd rev ed.). International Universities Press. (Original work published 1984)

Rubin, J. B. (1998). *A psychoanalysis for our time: Exploring the blindness of the seeing I*. New York University Press.

Rudnytsky, P. L. (1991). *The psychoanalytic vocation: Rank, Winnicott, and the legacy of Freud*. Routledge.

Sands, S. H. (1997). Self psychology and projective identification – Whither shall they meet? A reply to the editors (1995). *Psychoanalytic Dialogues, 7*, 651–668. https://doi.org/10.1080/10481889709539210

Shane, E. (2017). How Roger Frie and Ilene Philipson provide context for understanding Heinz Kohut: The man and his work. *Psychoanalysis, Self and Context, 12*(3), 244–252. https://doi.org/10.1080/24720038.2017.1320104

Siegel, A. (1996). *Heinz Kohut and the psychology of the self*. Routledge.

Slavin, M. O., & Kriegman, D. (1998). Why the analyst needs to change toward a theory of conflict, negotiation, and mutual influence in the therapeutic process. *Psychoanalytic Dialogues, 8*(2), 247–284. https://doi.org/10.1080/10481889809539246

Sprengnether, M. (2003). Mouth to mouth: Freud, Irma, and the dream of psychoanalysis. *American Imago, 60*(3), 259–284.

Stern, S. (2004). The yin and yang of intersubjectivity: Integrating self-psychological and relational thinking. In W. J. Coburn (Ed.), *Transformations in self psychology: Progress in self psychology* (Vol. 20, pp. 3–20). The Analytic Press/Taylor & Francis Group.

Strenger, C. (1989). The classic and the romantic vision in psychoanalysis. *The International Journal of Psychoanalysis, 70*(4), 593–610.

Strozier, C. B. (2001). *Heinz Kohut: The making of a psychoanalyst*. Farrar, Straus, and Giroux.

Strozier, C. B. (2018). *Heinz Kohut: The making of a psychoanalyst* (A. Pechler, Trans.). Carmel & The Israel Association for Self Psychology and the Study of Subjectivity. [Hebrew] (Original work published 2001)

Symington, N. (1993). *Narcissism: A new theory*. Karnac Books.

Togashi, K., & Kottler, A. (2021). From a cohesive self to a relational being: The evolution of the psychology of the self to the psychology of being human. *Psychoanalytic Inquiry, 41*(3), 187–198.

Widom, C. S., Czaja, S. J., & Paris, J. (2009). A prospective investigation of borderline personality disorder in abused and neglected children followed up into adulthood. *Journal of Personality Disorders, 23*(5), 433–446. https://doi.org/10.1521/pedi.2009.23.5.433

Winnicott, D. W. (1964). Review of C. G. Jung, memories, dreams, reflections. *The International Journal of Psychoanalysis, 45*, 450–455.

Winnicott, D. W. (1965). The maturational processes and the facilitating environment: Studies in the theory of emotional development. *The International Psychoanalytical Library, 64*, 1–276. The Hogarth Press and the Institute of Psycho-Analysis.

Winnicott, D. W. (1971). *Playing and reality*. Tavistock Publications.

Winnicott, D. W. (1988). *Human nature*. Routledge. https://read.amazon.com/?asin=B073RQG8L9&ref_=kwl_kr_iv_rec_11

Winnicott, D. W. (1990). *Deprivation and delinquency* (C. Winnicott, R. Shepherd, & M. Davis, Eds.). Routledge. (Original work published 1984)

Winnicott, D. W. (2018). *Psycho-analytic explorations* (C. Winnicott, R. Shepherd, & M. Davis, Eds.). Routledge. (Original work published 1989)

5 The attachment to the other

The theorists pushed to the margins

Introduction

The first chapter of this book discusses the underlying narcissistic bias common to the leading theorists of mainstream psychoanalysis, starting with Freud, Winnicott, and Kohut and continuing with other prominent theorists like Hartmann, Mahler, and Klein, who were primarily concerned with the self, presenting the other as an elusive entity – in particular, the mother as designed to serve the child, fulfilling various functions, important as they may be, while she stayed in the background. As noted, other voices were heard along the way that emphasized the fundamental centrality of interpersonal relationships per se in the human psyche. However, they were pushed to the margins by the psychoanalytic establishment of the time. Inter alia, the theorists known as neo-Freudians, among them Sullivan, Horney, Fromm, and Thompson, underscored the essential role of interpersonal relationships – as contrasted to instinctual drives – in human psychology and held that the individual could only be understood in the context of his interpersonal relationships and social environment. Those architects of the relational model had a far-reaching impact on psychoanalytic thought, shifting its focus toward relational and intersubjective perspectives, which have gained momentum since and are popular in contemporary psychoanalysis (as described in detail in the next chapter).

While the neo-Freudians as well as the intersubjective relational theorists attenuated the narcissistic bias in psychoanalytic theory by highlighting the role of interpersonal relationships and sociocultural factors in shaping the personality, they failed to place due emphasis on the unique emotional bond that forms between people in a close intimate relationship.[1] In view of this, I have chosen to focus on four influential, although previously marginalized theorists who highlighted the intrinsic importance of the primary parent-child emotional bond in psychological development and thus voiced a position that was the very antithesis of the narcissistically biased position of mainstream psychoanalysis – Sándor Ferenczi, Michael Balint, Ronald Fairbairn, and John Bowlby. Ferenczi can be crowned as the founding father of the intersubjective relational school, given his emphasis on the innate need for

DOI: 10.4324/9781003538295-5

interpersonal relatedness, in general, and intimate relationships of love and tenderness, in particular, and his contribution to the two-person psychology approach. Balint, who was Ferenczi's disciple and follower, believed in primary love, as opposed to the Freudian concept of primary narcissism, and underscored the fundamental role of a close emotional relationship between infant and mother in the psychic life of the infant. Fairbairn, a contemporary of Winnicott who lived and worked in Edinburgh independently of any psychoanalytic school, argued, based on his clinical work with children exposed to parental abuse or neglect who nevertheless clung to the abusive parent, that humans were primarily motivated by the search for relatedness with a significant other rather than by drive satisfaction, as maintained by Freud and his followers. Bowlby coined the term *affectional bond* to denote the deep emotional connection between individuals that organizes psychic life and laid the groundwork for a relational theory that has expanded and evolved since with significant implications for developmental psychology. Attachment theory, as labeled and formulated by Bowlby, is concerned with the primary emotional bond formed between infant and parent that is the model for subsequent affectional bonds formed in later stages of life.

Sándor Ferenczi (1873–1933)

Ferenczi was a close associate and friend of Freud and, for a time, his analysand. Yet he had mixed feelings about Freud. On the one hand, Ferenczi saw Freud as a revered father figure whose affection he sought and as a trusted confidant with whom he could consult on personal matters (specifically his relations with women). On the other hand, he was deeply disappointed by Freud's failure to recognize his professional contributions and resented his distant manner. Their lifelong relationship was thus characterized by ups and downs. It seems that Ferenczi's nonconformity and creative spirit – at times, too free-spirited – were incompatible with Freud's reserved, rigid, and authoritarian approach.

Looking for the therapeutic method that would best benefit his patients, Ferenczi tried out various clinical practices. He truly believed in straightforward and honest interpersonal relationships and specifically in more equal relationships between therapist and patient. Accordingly, he put to the test a mutual analysis technique whereby the analysand was a co-participant in a reciprocal therapeutic encounter (Ferenczi & Dupont, 1988):

> Certain phases of mutual analysis represent the complete renunciation of all compulsion and of all authority on both sides: they give the impression of two equally terrified children who compare their experiences, and because of their common fate understand each other completely and instinctively try to comfort each other.
>
> (p. 56)

Needless to say, Ferenczi's approach was at variance with the Freudian clinical practice, which assigned the analyst the role of the uninvolved knowledgeable figure of authority. Primarily concerned with the well-being of his patients, Ferenczi advocated self-disclosure of the analyst, even if it meant acknowledging his own weaknesses. His non-narcissistic, non-grandiose position in the therapeutic setting reflected his empathy for his patients and respect for their feelings. He believed that human goodness and compassion were innate, selfless qualities rather than defenses against antisocial instincts, yet noted that altruistic benevolence could only be expressed in the absence of early childhood pain and suffering. Thus, with reference to Freud's notion of reaction formation, Ferenczi suggested another source of such noble feelings:

> One comes to suspect that there is also a second source of mutual goodwill, more primary, natural, and nonneurotic. If we succeed in gaining insight into the psychic life of a child who as yet has been spared pain and suffering, then we come ultimately to the assumption that man becomes passionate and ruthless purely as a consequence of suffering. But if the child continues to live in an optimal environmental climate, then it is inclined (a) to share its own pleasure with the environment, (b) to take pleasure, without a feeling of envy, in development and wellbeing in the environment . . . It is therefore perhaps incorrect to attribute all manifestations of goodness or excessive goodness on the part of obsessional neurotics to compensated or overcompensated sadistic aggressiveness.
>
> (p. 151)

Ferenczi reiterated in his writings that children yearned for love – not for the fulfillment of their libidinal passion. He distinguished between the language of tenderness – appropriate for children – and the language of passion – the language of adults, which is inappropriate for children (Ferenczi, 1988). Ferenczi maintained, as originally suggested by Freud,[2] that mental disorders originated in real-life, traumatic sexual abuse in early childhood rather than in unconscious libidinal wishes and phantasies. The clinical practice adopted by Ferenczi reflected his belief that above all, patients needed an empathetic therapist who would love them and identify with their pain and suffering. In fact, he stated that the analyst's empathy and love for his patients were essential to the success of the psychoanalytic process. Thus, while Freud saw himself in the role of the analyst as a distant, neutral, father figure offering intellectualized interpretations, Ferenczi assumed the motherly role, offering his patients tenderness, emotional intimacy, sympathy, and identification. He disapproved of the preoccupation with transference in the therapeutic dialogue, whereby the analyst put himself at the center of attention as if he were the most important figure in the life of the patient and saw the excessive emphasis on the transference relationship as narcissistic.

In line with his non-narcissistic position and concern for the dignity of the vulnerable other, Ferenczi (Ferenczi, 1988; Ferenczi & Dupont, 1988) suggested that the sense of solidarity with the other, as reflected, inter alia, in social engagement and advocacy on behalf of vulnerable and marginalized populations (e.g., homosexuals and transvestites), was based on recognition of our mutual vulnerability, shared empathy, and innate human benevolence, over and above any self-seeking narcissistic interests.

However, the contribution of Ferenczi to psychoanalytic thought and practice was ignored and dismissed by Freud as well as by his followers and successors. Ernest Jones, a close colleague of Freud and an influential figure in the psychoanalytic establishment in the 1920s and 1930s, was apparently behind the rumor of Ferenczi's mental deterioration in his last years and the allegation that Ferenczi's final contributions were the product of his supposed insanity. Judith Dupont, who brought Ferenczi's writings to the public attention after more than five decades of censorship, observed[3] that any attempt by Ferenczi to make his voice heard provoked blatant rejection and that following his death, his works were suppressed and finally sentenced to oblivion (along with those of Otto Rank) by Jones in the third volume of his monumental biography of Freud. It should be noted, though, that while Ferenczi was marginalized due to his unorthodox views and practices, his failure to formulate a systematic theory and leave behind a complete corpus of writings further undermined his standing in mainstream psychoanalysis.

Michael Balint (1896–1970)

Balint was a disciple of Ferenczi and, to a large extent, his follower and successor. Like Ferenczi, Balint highlighted the fundamental significance of close emotional relationships, specifically the emotional bond between child and parent and its central role in healthy psychological development as well as the analyst-patient relationship in the clinical setting. In this context, Balint (1968/1979) noted, "The aim of all human striving is to establish – or, probably, re-establish – an all-embracing harmony with one's environment, to be able to love in peace" (p. 65).

Balint proposed a non-narcissistic "theory of primary relationship to the environment," that is, a theory of "primary love" (Balint, 1968/1979, p. 65) as a substitute for Freud's theory of primary narcissism.[4] According to Balint's theory of primary love, right from the moment of birth, the infant is attuned to the mother, whose love he needs and on whom he depends for the fulfillment of all his other needs. Yet while the infant desperately needs the love of the mother and craves intimacy and harmony with her, he still cannot perceive her as a separate object with feelings and wishes of her own:

> Lastly, it is worth remembering that our relationship to the air surrounding us has exactly the same pattern. We use the air, in fact we cannot live without it; we inhale it in order to take parts out of it and use them as we want; then, after putting substances into it that we want to get rid of, we exhale it – without paying the slightest attention to it. In fact, the air must be there for us, and as long as it is there in sufficient supply and quality, we do not take any notice of it. This kind of environment must simply be

> there, and as long as it is there – for instance, if we get enough air – we take its existence for granted, we do not consider it as an object, that is, separate from us; we just use it. The situation changes abruptly if the environment is altered – if, for instance, in the adult's case the supply of air is interfered with – then the seemingly uncathected environment assumes immense importance, that is, its latent true cathexis becomes apparent.
>
> (pp. 66–67)

However, as argued by Balint, in the absence of an adequate response to the needs of the infant, a "basic fault" is caused with a devastating impact on the budding psyche of the infant, a fault that can never be fully healed, not even through lengthy in-depth psychoanalysis.

As Balint (1968/1979) further argued, the relationship between analyst and patient has a crucial role in the healing of the basic fault, even though "it may amount only to a healing with defect" (p. 22). Balint stressed that the processes the patient was going through were directly influenced by the analyst, by the analyst's response to the patient, and by the nature of the relationship established by the analyst with the patient. That is, as per Balint, the psychoanalytic process is taking place between two people rather than within the mind of one person and thus concerns interpersonal aspects rather than just intrapsychic aspects. The relational two-person psychology, as Balint termed it, exceeds the boundaries of traditional one-person psychology since the experiential therapeutic relationship is in itself healing and, at times, even more so than verbal interpretations and insights. Thus, when words fail, "additional therapeutic agents should be considered . . . to inactivate the basic fault by creating conditions in which it can heal off." To that end, "the patient must be allowed to regress" to the area of the basic fault "before the patient can give up, very tentatively at first, his compulsive pattern" and "begin anew" (p. 166). The regressive process enables the patient to experience (once again), vis-à-vis the analyst, some sort of primary, primitive object relations and thereby get back to the area of the traumatic basic fault and heal it, although "its scar will remain for ever" (p. 183). The analyst, for his part, "should be willing to carry the patient, not actively but like water carries the swimmer or the earth carries the walker, that is, to be there for the patient, to be used without too much resistance against being used" (p. 167). The regression to the area of the traumatic basic fault fostered by the analyst to enable the establishment of experiential therapeutic relations with the patient was described by Balint as "the benign form of regression," as distinguished from "the malignant form of regression" – a term that he used to denote pathological defensive regression.

One of the known cases that illustrates Balint's clinical approach, according to which an effective analytic practice is not necessarily interpretive, is that of an analysand in her late twenties who felt stuck and unable to achieve anything in any area of life. In the course of the analytic treatment, it emerged that she was crippled by her fear to take risks and make decisions and that "apparently the most important thing for her was to keep her head safely up, with both feet firmly planted on the ground," as Balint (1968/1979) told her. When she mentioned in response that much as she had tried, she never managed to do a somersault, Balint suggested that she give it a try, "whereupon she got up from the couch and, to her great amazement, did a perfect somersault." As noted by Balint, it "proved to be a real breakthrough," achieved through the patient's acting out rather than following verbal interpretation, and it led to significant changes in her life (pp. 128–129).

Balint criticized the omnipotent position characteristic of traditional psychoanalysts and emphasized, like Ferenczi, the importance of the analyst's recognition of his own weaknesses. Also, like Ferenczi, Balint believed in innate human goodness and saw sadism, hate, and aggression as pathological phenomena stemming from an earlier state of deficiency, frustration, or trauma.

Along with the other precursors of the intersubjective relational school, Balint was marginalized for decades from the mainstream psychoanalytic discourse, and as he himself observed, "All these analysts, including myself, belong – not to the 'classical' massive centre – but to the fringe. We are known, tolerated, perhaps even read, but certainly not quoted" (Balint, 1968/1979, p. 155). His observation was echoed by Dupont,[5] who noted that like Ferenczi, Balint was sentenced to silence, ignored and unappreciated by his contemporaries.

Ronald Fairbairn (1889–1964)

Fairbairn lived and worked in Edinburgh, Scotland, far away from the heated controversy between the followers of Anna Freud and the supporters of Melanie Klein that divided the British Psychoanalytical Society in London of the early 1940s. Fairbairn developed a whole new theory that challenged and offered an alternative to Freudian drive theory. Fairbairn maintained that the libido was not pleasure oriented nor specifically seeking instinctual gratification, but rather driven by the quest for a close relationship with the other. His theory was based on his clinical work with children exposed to traumatic parental abuse and neglect who nevertheless were still clinging to the abusive parent. That is, although those parents failed to respond to the needs of their children or, even worse, actually hurt them, the children surprisingly showed a deep need to relate to and connect with their parents. According to Fairbairn, what children need above all is the love of their parents and a feeling of security and trust in their parents. When the parental figure rejects or frustrates the child, dissociation of the self occurs, which is designed to enable the child to maintain connection with the internalized image of the parent at any cost. This schizoid defensive splitting of the self, as conceptualized by Fairbairn, is reflected in the rejection of authentic relationships with real-life people and regression to imagined relationships with the internalized primary objects, while the pattern of those relationships is projected onto interpersonal relationships formed later on in life. Thus, for instance, the choice of a partner in couple relationships is often a choice of unrewarding, mentally painful relationships with an alienated, judgmental, violent, self-centered, depressive, or otherwise emotionally troubled or abusive partner. Trying as such relations may be, they provide a sense of familiarity and connection with the parental figure, no matter how frustrating or abusive that figure might have been, as well as hope for achieving the sought emotional intimacy that was absent in the early childhood relationship.

Furthermore, as noted by Fairbairn, it is not only the hope for a corrective experience and regained love that preserves the pattern of negative relationships experienced in infancy but also the fear of an emotional vacuum once the parental figure is abandoned, as it were, and the feelings of guilt, self-hate, and self-destruction that could arise following such desertion. Thus, rather than revolving around the Oedipal complex, the real intrapsychic drama concerns the emotional relationships between parents and their children and the mental pain attendant on the distance from and rejection by the parental figure. The anxiety of separation or loss is then, according to Fairbairn, the most fundamental anxiety rather than castration anxiety, as posited by Freud, or the anxiety of disintegration of the self, as suggested by Winnicott and Kohut.

Guntrip, who was an analysand of Fairbairn and his follower, highlighted and reiterated the centrality of close relationships – with the parental figures, in infancy and childhood, and with other significant figures, later on in life. In this context, Guntrip (1968/1992) pointed out the difference between Fairbairn and Winnicott in their conceptualization of infantile love:

> Fairbairn regards the destructive element in infantile 'love' or 'need of the object' as a direct reaction to rejection. Winnicott regards a destructive element in infantile 'need' as normal and natural. Here again it seems to me equivocal to use the same term 'love' for such different things.
>
> (p. 429)

The distinction made by Guntrip calls to mind the previously cited observation by Ferenczi (Ferenczi & Dupont, 1988) regarding the innate source of human goodness and compassion, which reflects his belief that love is not necessarily related to aggressiveness and destructiveness.

Like Ferenczi and Balint, Fairbairn maintained that the relationship between analyst and patient was essential to healing and in itself healing, no less so than intellectualized interpretations. Similarly, Fairbairn believed that the patient needed the analyst's love and sympathy. Yet the patient may be expected to experience the analyst at first the way he experiences the internalized primary objects and project onto the analyst his split-off negative parts (perceiving the analyst as cold and distant, e.g., 'the same as my mother, who rejected me'). The patient could thus fear getting close to the analyst lest he get hurt once again. It is only gradually that the patient's experience of the analyst may change, as he sees the analyst in a new, more positive light, "as a sufficiently good object" (Fairbairn, 1952/2001, p. 70), and it is then that his internalized object representations and pattern of relationships with significant figures in his adult life may change as well.

Fairbairn and his original ideas had a negligible impact on psychoanalytic theory and practice at the time. His contemporaries were not ready yet to give up the Freudian notion that humans were driven by the need for instinctual gratification and accept the idea suggested by Fairbairn that it was the quest for a close relationship with the other that motivated us humans. In this context. Ogden (2010) observed:

> To my mind, Fairbairn's theory of internal object relations constitutes one of the most important contributions to the development of analytic theory in its first century. Yet, judging from the scarcity of references to his work in the analytic literature, particularly in North American and Latin American writing, his theoretical ideas . . . and his clinical thinking . . . have attracted far less interest and study than have other major 20th century analytic theorists such as Klein, Winnicott and Bion.
>
> (p. 102)

Beyond the difficulty of embracing such a dramatic paradigm shift in psychoanalytic theory and practice, two other factors contributed to the marginalization of Fairbairn. First, his arcane language and obstruse theoretical concepts were too intricate to fathom and second, as noted, he lived and worked in Edinburgh, miles away from the British Psychoanalytical Society and its center of influence in London, and thus remained uninvolved in the psychoanalytic discourse of that era.

John Bowlby (1907–1990)

Bowlby's attachment theory places emotional attachment – and specifically the infant's emotional attachment to the parental figure, displayed from the very moment of birth – at the center of psychic life. Drawing on evolutionary theory, Bowlby ascribed the phenomenon of emotional attachment to the primal survival instinct of mammalian and avian species, in general, and human infants, in particular, as reflected in their seeking of proximity to an adult caregiver, who is looked to for support, safety, security, and protection from danger (e.g., protection from predators). Bowlby formulated his theory based on the extensive observations and research on the behavior of both humans and nonhuman species. He found the ethological studies of Konrad Lorenz of special interest, in particular, Lorenz's 1935 study of the imprinting behavior displayed by just hatched ducklings and goslings, who instinctively bonded with the first animate object they were exposed to, typically the mother figure, whom they followed everywhere, or even the researcher's foot, to which they tenaciously clung. As noted by Bowlby (1988), the study "showed that in some animal species a strong bond to an individual motherfigure could develop without the intermediary of food: for these young birds are not fed by parents but feed themselves by catching insects" (p. 25). Another well-known and frequently referenced study cited by Bowlby is the 1959 study of rhesus macaques by Harlow and Zimmermann, which likewise showed that the attachment of an infant to the parental figure was not necessarily contingent on feeding and that "infants show a marked preference for a soft dummy 'mother', despite its providing no food, to a hard one that does provide it" (p. 26). These are just two of the dozens of studies cited by Bowlby in his writings in support of his attachment theory.

Bowlby believed, like Fairbairn, that the anxiety of separation or loss was the most fundamental anxiety (rather than the anxiety of disintegration of the self or, for instance, guilt anxiety over taboo impulses). Bowlby similarly maintained that anger and aggressiveness were caused by parental rejection, detachment, or lack of love. It should be noted in this context that Bowlby (1988) highlighted the need for emotional intimacy not only between infant and parent and not merely as a developmental need in infancy but also as a fundamental need throughout life and as an indication of mental health:

> Within the attachment framework therefore intimate emotional bonds are seen as neither subordinate to nor derivative from food and sex. Nor is the urgent desire for comfort and support in adversity regarded as childish, as dependency theory implies. Instead the capacity to make intimate emotional bonds with other individuals, sometimes in the careseeking role and sometimes in the caregiving one, is regarded as a principal feature of effective personality functioning and mental health. (p. 121)

The ability to form mutual and rewarding interpersonal relationships in adulthood evidently depends on the primary emotional bond formed between infant and parent, which is internalized as a *working model* for significant affectional bonds formed later on in life. A secure emotional bond with the parental figures provides the child with a *secure base*, as termed by Bowlby, on which the child can rely and to which he can return when feeling stressed or distressed. On the other hand, an insecure attachment pattern (whether anxious-avoidant, dismissive-avoidant, ambivalent, or disorganized), whereby the attachment figure fails to provide the child with safety, security, and stability, is liable to give rise to an ambivalent relational pattern or, for instance, result in defensive avoidance of intimate relationships with the parent or with a significant other ('I don't need him . . . I can get along quite well on my own').

Bowlby explored in depth the issue of loss and grief, inter alia, in Volume 3 of his *Attachment and Loss* trilogy (Bowlby, 1980), reiterating the painful significance of separation from or loss of a loved one, the irreplaceability of the lost loved one, and the far-reaching implications of the separation or loss for the separated or bereaved. Bowlby's approach to the issue points to his non-narcissistic position and reflects his perception of the unique and fundamental relationship with a significant other. In the context of infant-parent relationships, Bowlby (1988) saw the broad picture – from the point of view of the infant as well as from the mother's perspective, taking into account the mother's personality, emotional needs, and fears as directly and indirectly affecting the infant and, furthermore, noting the need for emotional support not only for the infant but also for the mother. With reference to the clinical setting, Bowlby maintained that the role of the analyst was to serve as a *secure base* for the patient and thereby enable a corrective experience in his interaction with the patient while providing the patient with the conditions for exploring the internalized representations of his primary attachment patterns, ingrained over the years – this, with the aim of "restructuring them in the light of the new understanding he acquires and the new experiences he has in the therapeutic relationship" (p. 138).

Bowlby was criticized and derided by the psychoanalytic establishment of the time and even dismissed as unworthy of the title psychoanalyst. This negative attitude could be attributed to a number of factors, first and foremost, his emphasis on the fundamental centrality of real-life relationships in early childhood rather than on the phantasy worlds of children and adults, which were then considered the key to understanding the human psyche. Second, the empirical and, in particular, the ethological research basis of his theorizing was controversial in various ways and incompatible with the then prevailing ideas of psychoanalytic theory and practice Yet over the years, Bowlby's attachment theory has gained recognition, and it is currently considered a leading or, actually, the leading theory in the area of developmental psychology.

Notes

1 As noted, schizoid self-sufficiency, that is, the denial of the need for emotional attachment to and dependence on a significant other, is one of the core features of narcissism.
2 Freud subsequently changed position and presented his theory of infantile sexuality, which focused on the world of libidinal phantasies in infancy.
3 As cited in the preface to the 2006 Hebrew translation of Balint's (1968/1979) *The Basic Fault*.
4 Adopted by Winnicott and Kohut.
5 As cited in the aforementioned preface to the 2006 Hebrew translation of Balint's (1968/1979) *The Basic Fault*.

References

Balint, M. (1979). *The basic fault: Therapeutic aspects of regression*. Tavistock Publications. (Original work published 1968)

Balint, M. (2006). *The basic fault: Therapeutic aspects of regression* (H. Gilad, Trans.; O. Rosen, Trans. of Preface by Judith Dupont). Am Oved. [Hebrew] (Original work published 1968)

Bowlby, J. (1980). *Attachment and loss. Vol. 3: Loss, sadness and depression*. Basic Books.
Bowlby, J. (1988). *A secure base: Parent-child attachment and healthy human development*. Basic Books.
Fairbairn, W. R. (2001). *Psychoanalytic studies of the personality*. Routledge. (Original work published 1952)
Ferenczi, S. (1988). Confusion of tongues between adults and the child: The language of tenderness and of passion. *Contemporary Psychoanalysis*, *24*(2), 196–206.
Ferenczi, S., & Dupont, J. (Eds.). (1988). *The clinical diary of Sándor Ferenczi* (M. Balint & N. Z. Jackson, Trans.). Harvard University Press.
Guntrip, H. (1992). *Schizoid phenomena, object relations and the self*. Karnac Books. https://read.amazon.com/?asin=B005RX17FW&ref_=kwl_kr_iv_rec_15 (Original work published 1968)
Ogden, T. H. (2010). Why read Fairbairn? *The International Journal of Psychoanalysis*, *91*(1), 101–118. https://doi.org/10.1111/j.1745-8315.2009.00219.x

6 The relational intersubjective school

From the margins into the mainstream

Ferenczi, Balint, Fairbairn, and Bowlby as well as other previously marginalized theorists like Sullivan, Horney, Fromm, and Thompson who underscored the essential role in mental life of interpersonal relationships, whether between closely attached individuals or in the broader sociocultural context, have gained recognition in recent decades by theorists associated with the relational intersubjective school. Originating in the United States, the relational intersubjective school (for the sake of brevity, hereinafter referred to as the intersubjective school) is apparently the most influential and popular school in contemporary psychoanalysis. With the focus on interpersonal relationships as central to the human psyche, the intersubjective school is concerned with real-life human interactions as well as with internalized representations of primary attachment patterns. It encompasses a range of voices and diverse perspectives of various relational and intersubjective theorists, among them Robert Stolorow, Stephen Mitchell, Lewis Aron, Jessica Benjamin, Thomas Ogden, Donna Orange, and Owen Renik (Mitchell & Aron, 1999). Thus, for instance, while the intersubjective aspect of the encounter between analyst and analysand as two mutually interacting subjects is commonly highlighted by relational and intersubjective theorists and generally reflected in a rather informal clinical practice, including at times the analyst's self-disclosure, Ogden, who likewise viewed the analytic encounter as centrally involving the intersubjective field jointly created by the analytic pair – the *analytic third,* as he coined it – adopted a more traditional clinical approach advocating a certain distance between analyst and analysand as well as the analyst's anonymity. Given the wide range of views falling under the umbrella term *intersubjective*, the following discussion does not purport to specifically address the unique contribution or approach of each theorist associated with the intersubjective school. As noted, their diverse positions aside, all relational and intersubjective theorists share a common focus on the fundamental centrality of interpersonal relationships in the human psyche and emphasize the need for contextual consideration of psychic phenomena – with reference to the intersubjective contexts in which

DOI: 10.4324/9781003538295-6

they take place. This view has a solid theoretical and empirical basis (Blatt, 2008). Interpersonal relatedness is fundamental to human existence, both on the personal level of emotional attachment between individuals and on the more general social and cultural level. Tracing the evolvement of the idea of intersubjectivity, Aron (1996, p. 67) noted that the term was introduced into American psychoanalysis by Stolorow and his colleagues, who defined intersubjectivity theory as follows:

> Intersubjectivity theory is a field theory or systems theory in that it seeks to comprehend psychological phenomena not as products of isolated intrapsychic mechanisms, but as forming at the interface of reciprocally interacting subjectivities [Stolorow and Atwood, 1992, p. 1].

In the same spirit, Benjamin (1990) discussed the dynamics between two individuals seen as mutually interacting subjects. That is, Benjamin too maintained that the parties to a relationship cannot be considered separately, apart from the intersubjective context. Her discussion centered on their capacity for mutual recognition of each other's subjectivity. According to Benjamin, such mutual recognition, whereby each party recognizes the other as having "a separate and equivalent center of self" (p. 186) and a separate subjective world of feelings, needs, attitudes, and thoughts, reflects personality maturity and enables full enjoyment of the relationship. The interaction between two subjects who mutually recognize each other's subjectivity is in inherent conflict with a relationship described by Benjamin as narcissistic, which revolves around only one subject whose feelings and needs are at the center of attention while the other is seen as an object, serving as an extension or fulfilling a function. In this context, Benjamin criticized Mahler's separation-individuation theory, which highlighted the child's separation from the mother toward autonomy and the consolidation of self-identity while failing to duly consider the significance of the mother-child relationship per se as taking place between two subjects who recognize each other's subjectivity (the mother too needs to be recognized by her child) and who take pleasure in discovering each other's subjectivity. As noted by Benjamin, such mutuality between mother and child is not only enjoyable but also conducive to the consolidation of self-identity, no less so than the child's move toward separation, as "the child gains not only . . . independence (as traditionally emphasized) but also the pleasure of shared understanding" (p. 193).

The intersubjective perspective is reflected in the clinical setting, where the focus is on the encounter between the mutually interacting subjective worlds of analyst and analysand rather than on the analysand as a separate individual seen apart from the relational context. Thus, in contrast to the traditional psychoanalytic approach, the prevailing view in the intersubjective school is that the analyst's personality features and subjective world cannot and should not be ignored. Indeed, the analyst's presence is believed to have a significant role in the psychoanalytic situation. Specifically, as noted by

Aron (1991), the patient's experience of the analyst's subjectivity should be a central element of the analytic dialogue as such a dialogue is an essential part of the therapeutic process and a contributing factor to personal growth. While there are differences of opinion about the appropriate nature of the analyst's self-disclosure and related discourse with the analysand (e.g., should the analyst share with the analysand personal details or only thoughts and feelings that are directly related to the therapeutic encounter?), there is no question about the mutual influences of analyst and analysand in the encounter between the two, which should be taken into consideration to make sense of the processes that take place in the consulting room.

Intersubjectivity theory is primarily concerned with the therapeutic processes that occur in the clinical field, the therapeutic goals, and the role of the therapist, and less so with theoretical hypothesizing regarding universal human psychology. Thus, it has not presented consistent models of early childhood development, whether normal or pathological, nor suggested diagnostic criteria for personality pathology. It has likewise sidestepped theoretical conceptualizations of intrapsychic processes and structures and has not dealt with the etiology of specific symptoms. This may be attributed, in part, to the postmodern philosophy widely held by relational and intersubjective theorists, which questions the certainty and universality of objective truth, that is, truth that can be theoretically or empirically established and that is valid for all people. Rather, postmodernism emphasizes the multiplicity of truths, which are all seen as biased by personal perspectives and, as such, subjective and relative. Accordingly, any insight emerging in the therapeutic process is seen by relational and intersubjective theorists as jointly constructed by the analyst and analysand and thus reflecting their subjective narratives rather than as an objective truth discovered through bias-free enquiry. Furthermore, preconceived categories enforced on the patient are likewise considered biased and are thus shunned by relational and intersubjective theorists and practitioners. The more radical of them argue that there is no objective absolute truth whatsoever and that any position or statement is necessarily subject to individual perspective and therefore relative. The moderates among them believe that there are certain objective truths that should be taken into account but at the same time underscore their skepticism regarding universally applicable absolute truths. Their sweeping negation of absolute, universal truths illustrates how far psychoanalysis has moved away from the approach of Freud, reflected in his statement, *I don't believe in relativity, I believe in absolute truths* (Rolnik, 2019).

Intersubjectivity theory has also been considerably influenced by feminist ideas. In the spirit of equality advocated by feminism, intersubjectivity theory highlights the need for a more equal relationship between analyst and analysand and calls for a less hierarchical and less authoritative posture on the part of the analyst and for greater mutuality in the psychoanalytic situation, where the knowledgeable figure of authority who sees through the patient's mind and enforces his insights and interpretations on the patient has no longer a place. It is noteworthy that the issue at the center of intersubjectivity theory, that is, interpersonal relatedness and its crucial role in the human psyche, is perceived as closely associated with feminist values while the stereotypically masculine goals of separateness, independence, autonomy, and so on were for years the focal point of traditional psychoanalytic practice. Feminist thought has further contributed to a shift in perspective regarding the nature of the therapeutic encounter, which has come to be seen as occurring between two subjects, each with feelings, needs, and experiences of his own – this, in contrast to the traditional psychoanalytic view of the analyst-analysand relationship or, for that matter, the mother-child or woman-man relationship, as taking place between an indistinct object whose unique individuality was considered irrelevant and whose main role was need satisfaction and a subject whose needs had to be fulfilled.

Thus, after long years of marginalization, the groundbreaking ideas of Ferenczi have been brought to the forefront by the intersubjective school. In various respects, Ferenczi's non-narcissistic psychoanalytic approach is echoed in the wider contextual perspective taken by intersubjectivity theory and in its focus on the intersubjective and sociocultural contexts of human existence. Issues such as gender, sexual orientation, racism, cultural immigration, and social class have consequently been recognized as relevant to understanding the individual (Aron & Starr, 2013). Ferenczi's legacy is likewise reflected in the clinical practices adopted by the intersubjective school – specifically mutuality in the therapeutic setting, where the analyst is expected to acknowledge his limitations and assume an attentive and empathetic attitude with respect to the analysand, and the space allowed for expression of the analyst's subjectivity in the analytic dialogue (as advocated by various relational and intersubjective theorists and practitioners), which enables the analysand to deal with the notion of otherness rather than focus only on his own subjectivity. The intersubjective relationship between analyst and analysand, seen as a core element of the analytic dialogue, has significance even beyond the analytic situation, indicating the relevance of intersubjective exchange and reciprocal influences for all human relationships.

The narcissistic bias underlying intersubjectivity theory

Intersubjectivity theory has no doubt reduced the narcissistic bias in psychoanalysis by highlighting the fundamental centrality of interpersonal relationships in the human psyche and downgrading the status of authority of the know-it-all analyst. Yet the narcissistic bias is still reflected in various ways even in relational and intersubjective perspectives and clinical practices, as illustrated with reference to the three core features of narcissism discussed at length in Chapter 3 – grandiosity, schizoidism, and the difficulty acknowledging the otherness and separateness of the other.

Grandiosity

The analyst's omnipotence and exhibitionism

When it comes to the analytic situation, psychoanalysis, in general, is preoccupied with the here and now, focusing on the interchange between analyst and analysand while failing to pay due attention to mental content and processes that are not necessarily related to the therapeutic setting and the transference-countertransference relationship. The analyst is thus invested with disproportionate significance, as if he were the most important figure in the life of the analysand (Ferenczi & Dupont, 1988; Balint, 1968/1979). The intersubjective school has taken it even further, highlighting the analyst's presence and subjectivity in the analytic setting. However, the analyst's effort to establish himself as a separate subject in the analytic dialogue could be seen as intended to satisfy the analyst's own narcissistic needs (Aron, 1991). Moreover, some theorists and practitioners associated with the intersubjective school encourage the analyst's self-disclosure in a way that could push the analyst to focus on his own subjectivity and exhibitionistic needs at the expense of the analysand and his needs. While sharing with the analysand various aspects of the analyst's life, including feelings and personal details, should not be ruled out under certain circumstances, when serving as a means of achieving specific goals in the therapeutic process such as building trust relationships with the analysand or allowing the analysand to deal with the analyst's otherness, it should be done cautiously and sparingly. Yet some relational and intersubjective practitioners have taken it to the extreme. However, the often referenced argument regarding the analyst's irreducible subjectivity, highlighted in the title of Renik's (1993) paper, is misleading in my opinion. I believe that the analyst can and should tone down his presence and subjectivity and refrain from burdening the analysand with his personal concerns, needs, positions, and feelings, much like a parent who responds to his child's needs while putting aside his own personal affairs. Aron (1991) identified the danger of the analyst's narcissistic exhibitionism inherent in preoccupation with the analyst-analysand relationship and the analyst's subjectivity:

> The major problem for analysts in establishing themselves as subjects in the analytic situation is that because of their own conflicts they may abandon traditional anonymity only to substitute imposing their subjectivity on patients and thus deprive patients of the opportunity to search out, uncover, and find the analyst as a separate subject, in their own way and at their own rate . . . . Analysts' continuous interpretations of all material in terms of the patient-analyst relationship, as well as analysts' deliberate efforts to establish themselves as separate subjects, may be rightfully experienced as an impingement stemming from the analysts' own narcissistic needs.
>
> (p. 257)

It should be noted, though, that notwithstanding Aron's cautionary comments, he himself tended to encourage his analysands to deal with his subjectivity in the consulting room – unduly, it seems to me:

> In the clinical situation I often ask patients to describe anything that they have observed or noticed about me that may shed light on aspects of our relationship. . . . I encourage patients to tell me anything that they have observed and insist that there must have been some basis in my behavior for their conclusions. I often ask patients to speculate or fantasize about what is going on inside of me, and in particular I focus on what patients have noticed about my internal conflicts.
>
> (p. 252)

A case in point of the analyst's excessive self-disclosure is presented in a well-known paper by Davies (1994) presenting a clinical vignette of a young man who found it difficult to establish intimate relationships with women. Every romantic initiative by himself or the other side was cut short by his reserved, anxious, or even nauseated reaction. Tracing his difficulty to his shame and guilt over the complex, sexually tinged relationship he had experienced with his mother as a child, Davies sought to convince him that his seductive mother had a share in it too. At a certain point, Davies decided, as a "last resort" (p. 167), to disclose her sexual fantasies about him. While her self-disclosure was based on a therapeutic rationale, it shows how easily therapeutic boundaries can be violated, at times, at the service of the analyst's narcissistic needs, and thus lead down a slippery slope, to the detriment of the analysand.

Based on relational and intersubjective perspectives, the analyst may be led to believe that his presence in the consulting room in itself can make a difference and that "the analytic interaction totally organizes the patient's mind" (Eagle, 2003, p. 416). The patient's, and by the same token, the individual's intrapsychic reality is thus perceived as ephemeral and constantly changing along with the intersubjective context rather than as having a stable and enduring mental structure and content (Giovacchini, 2005; Mills, 2005). In this context, Eagle (2003, p. 416) cited Meissner as critically observing,

> It seems odd . . . that one would think of the patient, as he enters the consulting room for the first time, as without a history entirely of his own, without a developmental background, without a psychology and personality that he has acquired and developed in the course of a lifetime, all accomplished before he had any contact with the analyst. [Meissner, 1998, p. 422]

Excessive modesty – The other side of the coin

The narcissistic split between two extreme self-states, grandiosity, on the one hand, and a sense of imperfection and inferiority, on the other hand, is reflected in a way on the theoretical level as well. Thus, the postmodern position adopted by various relational and intersubjective theorists and practitioners that no absolute truth can be discovered about the human psyche or the patient's mind seems to reflect excessive modesty – the very opposite of the grandiose posture of authority that characterized psychoanalysts for years (Aron, 1991). Orange (2011) underscored the need for the analyst to recognize the limits of his knowledge, engage in a nonauthoritarian dialogue with the patient, and "acknowledge the experiential uncertainty of practice." In this context, Orange observed:

> An expert is a person who possesses a body of knowledge not readily accessible to the public and who is consulted, either on television or in private, for this expertise. One may have expert knowledge of a foreign political system, of a rare form of cancer, or of the intricacies of tax law. The psychoanalytically oriented clinician, on the contrary, is a practitioner whose expertise consists in Aristotelian *phronesis* (practical wisdom) regarding the emotional life of human beings. This wisdom is not a body of knowledge but a capacity for applied understanding of individual human beings in relational contexts.
>
> (p. 24)

As noted by Orange, the analyst is urged not to take himself too seriously and to remain a humble hermeneut. However, the position presented by Orange plays down the professional knowledge and expertise acquired by analysts based on long years of theoretical research, empirical studies, clinical practice, and their own extensive experience with a variety of patients. It ignores the gap between the experts, who have a deep knowledge of human psychology and the tools to understand the patient's mental world, and their patients, who are not necessarily familiar with mental phenomena and processes, whether conscious or unconscious. I believe that the radical position adopted by Orange is defensive and intended to offset the analyst's likely arrogance and grandiosity. Eagle (2003) pointed to the grandiosity underlying the apparently humble position of the analyst. Taking a different perspective, Eagle observed that the therapeutic goals set by relational and intersubjective theorists, in general, that is, "the creation of meaning systems and narratives" and "the organization and reorganization of experience" in collaboration with the patient, were no less grandiose than the goal of uncovering repressed objective truths sought by traditional psychoanalysis:

> Why would anyone object to this seemingly new humility and increasing democratization of the analytic relationship? There are a number of answers to this question. For one thing, I do not see any less arrogance in the claim that one is an expert in meaning making and the organization and reorganization of experience than in the traditional claim that one is an expert in reading unconscious wishes, motives, and defenses. Indeed, I find the latter more modest.
>
> (p. 418)

The world of fantasy, unconstrained by objective reality

As noted, postmodern epistemology, on which intersubjectivity theory draws to a large extent, rejects any possibility of objective knowledge that is independent of the observer's perspective. The more radical of relational and intersubjective theorists and practitioners thus maintain that no absolute truth can be discovered through psychoanalysis. Rather, the material emerging in the therapeutic discourse is seen as jointly constructed by the analyst and analysand based on their subjective narratives, and hence as reflecting a subjective reality. This line of thought represents a narcissistic position whereby the world of fantasy subjectively created by the partners to the analytic dialogue takes the place of objective reality. According to Bell (2009), it is a world "freed from the constraints of reality, a world where claims can never (by definition) be right, and so can never be wrong . . . a world of infinite possibility" (p. 344), where no choice has to be made among the myriad possibilities as all choices are equally right. Likewise, there is no need to cope with imperfection as the illusion of self-perfection "is superseded in postmodernism by the illusion of infinite freedom" (p. 340). The intersubjective school's conceptualization of the diversity of the self, as distinguished from the singleness of the self, reflects another facet of the narcissistic position – the wish to cast off all limitations of self-definition, "the inevitable limitations of being human" (p. 341). The point is illustrated in Chapter 3 with reference to a patient of mine who was enraged when I mentioned a behavior pattern of hers (her tendency to assume the role of the funny clown in unfamiliar social settings) as she apparently experienced her characterization in terms of specifically defined personality traits, like any common human, rather than as an amorphous, grandiose, godlike being without boundaries, as limiting and devaluing (Bach, 1985).

Schizoidism

The therapeutic focus on the development and enrichment of the individual's subjectivity

While intersubjectivity theory focuses on interpersonal relationships as central to the human psyche, the prime goal of psychoanalysis is seen as the development, enrichment, and diversification of the individual's experience of subjectivity. At the same time, life outside the therapeutic setting and real-life interpersonal relationships are not given due attention in the consulting room. In this context, Ogden (2004a) observed:

> The analytic situation, though in many ways unstructured, also has a quality of directionality that is derived from the fact that psychoanalysis most fundamentally is a therapeutic enterprise with the goal of enhancing the patient's capacity to be alive to as much as possible of the full spectrum of human experience. Coming to life emotionally is, to

> my mind, synonymous with becoming increasingly able to dream one's experience, which is to dream oneself into existence.
>
> (p. 864)

In the same spirit, Mitchell (1993) saw psychoanalysis as aimed at "fashioning a personal reality that feels authentic and enriching." Yet in the same breath Mitchell qualified his words, noting, "This goal does not suggest that contemporary psychoanalysis is individualistic and narcissistic, valuing only private meaning and concerns at the expense of connections to others and society at large" (p. 21). However, given that as suggested, the focus of psychoanalysis is on creating an authentic and enriching personal reality for the patient, it seems to be a definitely narcissistic schizoid goal centered on the self and the development of the self. But should it really be the overarching goal of the psychoanalytic process? Why not set as a primary goal the enhancement of the patient's capacity to establish close interpersonal relationships? And what about strengthening the patient's resilience and ability to cope with challenges and crises, or, for that matter, enabling him to acknowledge and accept his flaws, disabilities, or painful losses? I believe that an authentic, enriched, and vital self is not necessarily more mentally healthy although authenticity, vitality, and enrichment of the self are no doubt conducive to mental well-being. As noted in Chapter 3, creative and vital individuals can have mental problems in other significant spheres of life. Thus, they may have difficulty in forming emotionally intimate relationships or in constructively coping with reality or, in severe cases, they may even display defective reality testing.

The therapeutic setting as a glass bubble

The psychoanalytic setting has been fashioned over the years as a glass bubble, so to speak, where a potential space (to use Winnicott's terminology) is allowed for in-depth processes that cannot take place in casual encounters or common conversations on mundane affairs. The enclosed setting of the consulting room, isolated from the outside world, thus has a highly significant role in the therapeutic process. It encourages free association (an unstructured discourse); inspires profound consideration of deep-seated mental content, emotions, phantasies, dreams, unconscious needs, and so on; enables clinical interventions related to the transference-countertransference dynamics; and provides a stable framework (place and time schedule) for the analytic sessions. However, depending on the thickness of the glass bubble walls, that is, the extent to which it is separated from the outside world, this cocoon-like therapeutic setting could induce a shift toward narcissistic schizoid isolation from everything that occurs outside the consulting room – a "session-centric" tendency, as Wachtel (2009, p. 167) critically labeled it. I would rather suggest the term "malignant" glass bubble, in contrast to "benign" glass bubble (borrowing from Balint's concepts of benign and malignant forms of regression) – the latter denoting a therapeutic setting that supports fundamental

mental processes without totally shutting off reality. The approach adopted by relational and intersubjective theorists varies along the spectrum. Thus, for instance, Ogden (1989, 2004b) believes that there is no merit in collecting information about the patient at the beginning of the therapeutic process and no interest in details such as his age, marital status, number of children, if any, clinical symptoms, or even formative life events. Instead, his focus is on the way the patient presents himself as well as on the communication with the patient during the analytic encounter, which, as per Ogden, should be based to a large extent on the analyst's reverie and less so on conscious discourse related to objective, real-life content. While other theorists associated with the intersubjective school opt for a less associative and more structured discourse, they too focus the analytic dialogue on the intersubjective therapeutic encounter, the inner world of the patient, and the role of imagination and fantasy in creating and shaping reality rather than on real-life events and life reality.

The failure to highlight the phenomenon of emotional attachment

While intersubjectivity theory highlights the fundamental centrality of interpersonal relationships in the human psyche, it fails to place due emphasis on the unique phenomenon of emotional attachment, which should be distinguished from more or less close interpersonal relationships in general. Bowlby (1988) underscored the point, noting the distinction between relationships characterized by a deep emotional bond and social relations with no emotional attachment:

> Exploring the environment, including play and varied activities with peers, is seen as a third basic component and one antithetic to attachment behaviour. When an individual (of any age) is feeling secure he is likely to explore away from his attachment figure.
>
> (p. 121)

Bowlby defined emotional attachment as reflected primarily in a tendency to look for proximity to the attachment figure when feeling anxious or emotionally distressed; in extreme mental pain in reaction to separation, emotional distancing, abandonment, or loss; and in a sense of emptiness that cannot be filled upon the loss of an irreplaceable significant attachment figure. A wider perspective of the concept is suggested in this book, whereby emotional attachment does not necessarily involve a comforting attachment figure to whom one turns when in distress but is rather characterized by an intimate and unique emotional bond that is irreplaceable, whether or not it serves as a source of support and emotional security, for instance, the deep emotional bond between siblings or parents' affection for their children.

Cortina and Liotti (2010) distinguished, like Bowlby, between relationships that involved attachment to significant figures and social relationships in general. In their study of the different evolutionary origins of attachment and intersubjectivity, they argued that attachment was a fundamental phenomenon that preceded the development of intersubjectivity, that is, the capacity of the parties to a relationship to acknowledge the subjectivity of each other. Indeed, as noted by the authors, ethological studies show that attachment behavior is displayed by both humans and nonhuman species in the very early stages of life, while intersubjective abilities are progressively developed by humans but are found only to a limited extent in some animal species. Lorenz's study of the greylag goose's emotional reaction to the disappearance of a partner, cited by Fraley and Shaver (Cassidy & Shaver, 1999/2016), illustrates the fundamental nature of the phenomenon of attachment:

> The first response to the disappearance of the partner consists in the anxious attempt to find him again. The goose moves about restlessly by day and night, flying great distances and visiting all places where the partner might be found, uttering all the time the penetrating trisyllabic long-distance call. . . . The searching expeditions are extended farther and farther, and quite often the searcher himself gets lost, or succumbs to an accident. . . . All the objectively observable characteristics of the goose's behaviour on losing its mate are roughly identical with those accompanying human grief.
>
> (p. 40)

Further evidence of the fundamental significance of emotional attachment was provided by animal studies cited by Dozier and Rutter (Cassidy & Shaver, 1999/2016) that demonstrated the intense reaction of nonhuman primate and rodent young to separation from a primary attachment figure. Thus, it was found that "infant squirrel monkeys never habituated to separations from their mothers" and displayed "neuroendocrine distress responses to the separations." In another study, Harlow found that monkeys separated from their mother in infancy showed odd behavior as adults. "Most did not mate . . . and most that did mate showed very inappropriate parenting behaviors" (p. 696). And as might be expected, it has been extensively shown that children who were separated from their parents and grew up in institutions presented severe symptoms, both physically and mentally, although their various needs were fulfilled by substitute caregivers. The acute distress caused by separation from a primary attachment figure has no parallel in the context of intersubjective relationships.

The failure of intersubjectivity theory to highlight the fundamental significance of the phenomenon of attachment is also reflected in its focus on the temporary and transient. As noted, the theory allows for no stability of mental structure, and the individual's intrapsychic reality is perceived as changing along with the intersubjective context, which in turn changes with the status of the self – this, in contrast to attachment, which is by definition a stable, unchanging bond. Yet as observed in the next chapter, a shift of trend is evident not only in relational and intersubjective perspectives but across the field, as reflected in recent psychoanalytic views on loss and grief processes and in the growing awareness of the unique nature of the bond with a specific other and irreplaceability of a lost one.

The difficulty acknowledging the otherness and separateness of the other

There seems to be no question that intersubjectivity theory acknowledges and respects the other, the outsider, and the stranger (Orange, 2011), and hence allows a place for cultural and social diversity and stands out against bias targeting disadvantaged population groups (Aron & Starr, 2013). At the same time, certain theoretical conceptualizations and clinical practices point to the contrary, as shown next.

The amorphous, fluid self

The self is conceptualized in intersubjectivity theory as amorphous, fluid, variable, and diverse, without a stable, clearly defined structure or unique dynamics. The goal set for the therapeutic process is thus the development of the patient's subjectivity rather than the development of the patient's self – where the term *self* denotes an autonomous, separate entity with clear boundaries that can be observed as such (as conceptualized by Kohut and Kernberg, among others). Since the patient's experience of the self is seen as influenced to a large extent by the intersubjective context and as highly variable, the patient's unique identity is blurred. And it is not only the unique intrapsychic dynamics and distinctive personality traits of the patient that are blurred and disregarded but also his otherness and separateness in the clinical situation. Instead, relational and intersubjective theorists and practitioners tend to focus on the intersubjective field of shared thoughts, experiences, fantasies, and emotions jointly created by the analyst and patient – the *analytic third*, as coined by Ogden (1994, 2004). Mills (2005) criticized the focus on this intersubjective field, which blurred the boundaries between analyst and patient. Specifically, Mills critically noted the way Stolorow, Atwood, and their colleagues saw the intersubjective field – as an entity of its own at the center of the analytic process – while failing to focus on the patient as a separate other.

Uniform clinical practices and goals

When the patient is seen as a unique and separate individual with a distinct personality structure, specific mental conflicts, special needs, and so on, the clinical practice can be adapted to the patient's needs, and long-term goals can be set accordingly for the therapeutic process (McWilliams, 2011). Such personalization requires flexibility on the part of the analyst. However, intersubjectivity theory, in general,[1] sets preconceived therapeutic goals that do not necessarily meet the needs or wishes of each patient and thereby shows disregard for the otherness and separateness of the other. As noted, developing, enriching, and diversifying the patient's experience of subjectivity, creating an emotionally authentic personal reality, enhancing inner vitality, and promoting the capacity for engagement in intersubjective relationships are all worthy goals, alas, they are too general and indefinite to effectively respond to specific individual needs. Similarly, the style of intervention has to be adapted to the patient's personality, his developmental stage, and the phase of the therapeutic process. In line with intersubjectivity theory, Mitchell (1993) offered a generalized clinical approach that ignores the need for tailoring the clinical practice to the patient's unique needs:

> What the patient needs is not clarification or insight so much as a sustained experience of being seen, personally engaged, and, basically, valued and cared about. The "objective" interpretation, the very curative agent in the classical model, can in this view become the instrument for a repetition of the original trauma. Rather, what today's analysis provides is the opportunity to freely discover and playfully explore one's own subjectivity, one's own imagination.
>
> (p. 25)

However, while playful exploration may suit certain patients or the same patient at different stages of the psychoanalytic process, other patients may better benefit from intellectualized interpretations and insights or from any other personally adapted clinical practice.

The patient's life outside the therapeutic setting

Given the analyst's focus on the intersubjective relationship in the clinical situation and preoccupation with the here and now, not much room is left for consideration of the patient's life outside the therapeutic setting or mental processes that are not directly related to the analytic dialogue but have a central significance in his mental world.

Note

1 There are exceptions, of course. For instance, Renik believes that specific goals should be set for the therapeutic process in light of the patient's needs.

References

Aron, L. (1991). The patient's experience of the analyst's subjectivity. In S. A. Mitchell & L. Aron (Eds.), *Relational psychoanalysis: The emergence of a tradition* (pp. 243–268). Routledge.

Aron, L. (1996). *A meeting of minds: Mutuality in psychoanalysis*. The Analytic Press. https://read.amazon.com/?asin=B0B9KHXHZ1&ref_=kwl_kr_iv_rec_1

Aron, L., & Starr, K. (2013). *A psychotherapy for the people: Toward a progressive psychoanalysis*. Routledge/Taylor & Francis Group.

Bach, S. (1985). *Narcissistic states and the therapeutic process*. Jason Aronson.
Balint, M. (1979). *The basic fault: Therapeutic aspects of regression*. Tavistock Publications. (Original work published 1968)
Bell, D. (2009). Is truth an illusion? Psychoanalysis and postmodernism. *The International Journal of Psychoanalysis, 90*(2), 331–345. https://doi.org/10.1111/j.1745-8315.2009.00136.x
Benjamin, J. (1990). Recognition and destruction: An outline of intersubjectivity. In S. A. Mitchell & L. Aron (Eds.), *Relational psychoanalysis: The emergence of a tradition* (pp. 181–210). Routledge.
Blatt, S. J. (2008). *Polarities of experience: Relatedness and self-definition in personality development, psychopathology, and the therapeutic process*. American Psychological Association.
Bowlby, J. (1988). *A secure base: Parent-child attachment and healthy human development*. Basic Books.
Cassidy, J., & Shaver, P. R. (Eds.). (2016). *Handbook of attachment: Theory, research, and clinical applications* (3rd ed.). Guilford Press. https://read.amazon.com/?asin=B01F9KHK4Y&ref_=kwl_kr_iv_rec_2 (Original work published 1999)
Cortina, M., & Liotti, G. (2010). Attachment is about safety and protection, intersubjectivity is about social understanding and sharing: The relationship between attachment and intersubjectivity. *Psychoanalytic Psychology, 27*(4), 410–441. https://doi.org/10.1037/a0019510
Davies, J. D. (1994). Love in the afternoon: A relational reconsideration of desire and dread in the countertransference. *Psychoanalytic Dialogues, 4*(2), 153–170.
Eagle, M. N. (2003). The postmodern turn in psychoanalysis: A critique. *Psychoanalytic Psychology, 20*(3), 411–424.
Ferenczi, S., & Dupont, J. (Ed.). (1988). *The clinical diary of Sándor Ferenczi* (M. Balint & N. Z. Jackson, Trans.). Harvard University Press.
Giovacchini, P. (2005). Subjectivity and the ephemeral mind. In J. Mills (Ed.), *Relational and intersubjective perspectives in psychoanalysis: A critique*. Jason Aronson/Rowman & Littlefield.
McWilliams, N. (2011). *Psychoanalytic diagnosis: Understanding personality structure in the clinical process* (2nd ed.). Guilford Press.
Mills, J. (2005). A critique of relational psychoanalysis. *Psychoanalytic Psychology, 22*(2), 155–188. https://doi.org/10.1037/0736–9735.22.2.155
Mitchell, S. A. (1993). *Hope and dread in psychoanalysis*. Basic Books.
Mitchell, S. A., & Aron, L. (Eds.). (1999). *Relational psychoanalysis: The emergence of a tradition*. Routledge.
Ogden, T. H. (1989). *The primitive edge of experience*. Jason Aronson.
Ogden, T. H. (1994). The analytic third: Working with intersubjective clinical facts. *The International Journal of Psychoanalysis, 75*(1), 3–19.
Ogden, T. H. (2004a). The analytic third: Implications for psychoanalytic theory and technique. *The Psychoanalytic Quarterly, 73*(1), 167–195. https://doi.org/10.1002/j.2167-4086.2004.tb00156.x
Ogden, T. H. (2004b). This art of psychoanalysis: Dreaming undreamt dreams and interrupted cries. *The International Journal of Psychoanalysis, 85*(4), 857–877. https://doi.org/10.1516/D6R2-9NGF-YFJ2-5QK3
Orange, D. M. (2011). *The suffering stranger: Hermeneutics for everyday clinical practice*. Routledge.
Renik, O. (1993). Analytic interaction: Conceptualizing technique in light of the analyst's irreducible subjectivity. *Psychoanalytic Quarterly, 62*(4), 553–71.
Rolnik, E. (2019). *Sigmund Freud – Letters*. Modan. [Hebrew]
Wachtel, P. L. (2009). Knowing oneself from the inside out, knowing oneself from the outside in – The "Inner" and "Outer" worlds and their link through action. *Psychoanalytic Psychology, 26*(2), 158–170. https://doi.org/10.1037/a0015502

7 Loss and grief processes

A mini-theory shift

Introduction

The emergence of the intersubjective school[1] inspired a paradigm shift in psychoanalysis, in general, as its focus shifted toward relational and intersubjective perspectives, variously manifested in different psychoanalytic fields. Thus, Kohut's theory of self psychology evolved over the years, with a growing emphasis on the relational aspect of key concepts and processes, for instance, the twinship concept, increasingly seen as denoting a relational experience involving others rather than as focused merely on "the building of a cohesive self" (Togashi & Kottler, 2021, p. 187). Also noteworthy is the transition of post-Kohut self psychology from a one-person to a two-person psychology and redefinition of the analyst's role as a subject interacting with the analysand in a mutual, intersubjective relationship rather than as just an object (selfobject) fulfilling the analysand's narcissistic needs (Magid et al., 2021). It should be noted that the shift toward less narcissistic perspectives in various psychoanalytic fields has been inspired by other factors besides the emerging intersubjective school, including theoretical development and evolution in each field separately.

The efforts in recent decades to bridge the gap between psychoanalytic ideas and attachment theory, whether with reference to specific issues (Mitchell, 2000/2023; Diamond, 2004) or through an extensive, in-depth exploration of both the disagreements between attachment theory and psychoanalysis and their common foundations (Fonagy, 2001/2018), point to a growing recognition of the centrality of close interpersonal relationships in the organization of the human psyche. Other factors have also contributed to the toned-down narcissistic bias in contemporary psychoanalysis. Thus, the increasing psychoanalytic openness to other disciplines (philosophy, sociology, neurology, etc.) as well as the current emphasis on the significance of cultural factors for psychoanalytic theory, in general, and clinical practice, in particular (Harlem, 2009) reflect a clearly non-narcissistic position acknowledging the otherness of the other. Furthermore, an extensive research and clinical infrastructure has been developed that enriched the knowledge available in diverse areas and specifically in the area of infant development. In this

DOI: 10.4324/9781003538295-7

latter context, it has been shown that already in the very early stages of life, infants are engaged in a relational matrix, whereby the other is perceived as a separate object and subject rather than as merely a need fulfilling selfobject (Beebe & Lachmann, 2002).

To illustrate the shift toward a less narcissistic, more relational psychoanalysis, I have chosen to focus in this chapter on the specific issue of loss and grief processes, and not by chance. Recent psychoanalytic views on loss and grief processes reflect a growing awareness of the unique emotional bond with an irreplaceable significant other, indicating a distinctly non-narcissistic position. Since the present discussion concerns a specific shift of trend, it is referred to herein as a mini-theory shift. The related theoretical developments in recent decades reflecting a new emphasis on interpersonal relationships, in general, and on emotional attachment to a significant other, in particular, and hence the reduction of the narcissistic bias in psychoanalysis are described next.

The lifelong bonding with a departed loved one

As noted, in the extensively referenced essay *Mourning and Melancholia,* Freud (1917) described mourning as a process that normally came to an end with the withdrawal of the libido from the lost object of love (decathexis) and its displacement to a significant other. Later on, Freud (1923) presented a somewhat different view of mourning, suggesting that the conclusion of a normal mourning process involved the mourner's identification with the deceased and the internalization of the deceased's image in the mourner's ego, a process initially seen by Freud (1917) as indicative of pathological depression, that is, melancholia. However, while according to Freud's modified view of mourning, the process did not necessarily involve complete emotional detachment from the deceased, the deceased was not perceived as a separate entity with whom an internalized complex emotional relationship was maintained but rather as indistinguishably merged with the mourner's ego. The loss was not experienced, then, through feelings of grief over or longing for the departed loved one, memories of him, or imaginal dialogues with him, as would have been the case had the mourner maintained a continuing bond with the deceased. Thus, in either version of Freud's conceptualization of mourning, the process was actually seen as finally resolved through ultimate emotional detachment from the deceased and the intimate relationship experienced with him. It is noteworthy that notwithstanding Freud's own painful personal losses, specifically the agonizing loss of both his beloved daughter Sophie and her son, his cherished grandson Heinele, who succumbed to tuberculosis a couple of years afterward, and although Freud acknowledged that there could be no consolation for the loss of a dearly loved one and that no substitute could fill the gap,[2] he did not revise his theory of mourning. His approach to the issue of bereavement and mourning resounded for years in the psychoanalytic discourse (Gaines, 1997), influencing generations of practitioners and leading them to expect the normal resolution of the mourning process through the mourner's complete emotional detachment from the deceased or else regard the mourning process as pathological. In this spirit, Deutsch (1937) observed:

> The process of mourning as reaction to the real loss of a loved person *must be carried to completion*. As long as the early libidinal or aggressive attachments persist, the painful affect continues to flourish, and vice versa, the attachments are unresolved as long as the affective process of mourning has not been accomplished.
>
> (p. 21)

Yet the belief that the mourner's complete emotional detachment from the deceased can indeed be attained and that the mourning process can thus be carried to completion reflects a failure to recognize the fundamental significance of the deep and unique emotional bond with a dearly loved person, who cannot be replaced, not even by any significant other who may provide the needs previously provided by the departed loved one.

Kohut (1977, 1991/2011), for one, maintained that anyone was replaceable, as long as a substitute figure could provide the narcissistic functions provided by the lost object (as Kohut put it). Kohut's followers and successors in the self psychology school likewise held that a departed loved one could be replaced by anyone capable of fulfilling the same functions for the self, and thus carried on the trend minimizing the significance of the mourner's unique relationship with the deceased.

Thus, Shelby (1994) observed (as cited by Hagman, 2016, p. 74), "The central figures are not so much the mourner and the deceased as the mourner and the selfobject environment." That is, the focus as per Shelby should be on the self and the changes in the mourner's self following the selfobject loss rather than on the mourner's continuing bond with the deceased. His position is in line with Freud's (1923) later view of the conclusion of the mourning process as involving the internalization of the deceased's image in the mourner's ego, and hence as affecting the mourner's self. Kohut's successors highlighted this latter aspect of the mourning process as reflected, inter alia, in the adverse impact of the object loss on the mourner's self-worth and self-cohesion, which, as they argued, could be offset by a substitute selfobject replacing the lost object (Hagman, 1995; Palombo, 1982; Shelby, 1994). It should be noted, though, that following the recent shift in the psychoanalytic approach to loss and grief processes, the unique, irreplaceable continuing bond with the deceased has been increasingly recognized as an inseparable part of a normal mourning process even by theorists associated with the self psychology school. At the same time, excessive attention is given to the changes in the mourner's self and the significant role of a substitute selfobject in this context. Thus, for instance, George Hagman, a theorist and therapist who draws to a large extent on self psychology concepts and who has been for years engaged in exhaustive theoretical research and clinical practice in the area of bereavement, mourning, and grief, is well aware of the mourner's unique continuing bond with the departed loved one and its place as part of a normal mourning process[3] as well as of the need to distinguish between mourning as focused on the loss of this unique bond and mourning as primarily concerned with the changes in the mourner's self following the loss. Yet his writings deal mostly with the changes in the mourner's self due to the loss of a selfobject rather than with the loss of a significant other perceived as a separate and unique object and its meaning for the mourner. Hagman (1995) provided the following explanation for his choice of focus:

> Unfortunately, the nature of the focus of this chapter does not allow a complementary discussion of mourning for the lost object as an object in its own right, apart from its selfobject functions. The highlighting of the transmuting internalization of selfobject functions does not mean to imply that the experience of "object loss" is not important – far from it. However, over the years the psychoanalytic literature has dealt extensively with the problem of object loss, and my goal here is to explore an area that has been neglected.
>
> (p. 120)

Hagman thus devoted his 1995 discussion to the mourning process as inducing changes in the self through transmuting internalization of selfobject functions. That is, rather than dealing with the unique emotional relationship maintained with the lost object as an object in its own right, Hagman focused on the functional role of the selfobject and the changes in the mourner's self-structure generated in the absence of the selfobject. Hagman argued, and rightly so, that the psychoanalytic literature dealt extensively with the issue of object loss while neglecting the issue of selfobject loss, and thus freed himself from further consideration of the mourning process from the perspective of the loss of a separate, unique object. However, it should be noted that by and large, the psychoanalytic literature played down the significant and unique relationship with the departed dear one, even when referring to the deceased as a separate object in its own right. This is reflected, above all, in the traditional view that complete emotional detachment from the deceased is actually possible and that the mourning process can and must be carried to completion upon the replacement of the deceased by a substitute figure or otherwise, with the internalization of the deceased's image in the mourner's ego. In fact, over the years, the psychoanalytic discussion of the issue of mourning focused on the dimension of self-definition while neglecting the dimension of relatedness, to use the terminology of Blatt (2008). Concerned mainly with the dimension of self-definition, Hagman (1995) believes that psychoanalytic therapy should focus on the changes in the mourner's self and the restoration of the self following the loss rather than on the mourner's continuing bond with the deceased, although he does acknowledge the mourner's enduring emotional attachment to the deceased:

> From the perspective of self psychology, the goal of mourning is the restoration of the self after the rupture of a primary selfobject bond. . . . In the treatment of the bereaved, the focus of analysis should be on the person's struggle to repair, sustain, and regulate the self subsequent to the rupture of a crucial selfobject bond. The goal of mourning is not decathexis, but the retention of the lost selfobject functions through transformation of self-structure.
>
> (p. 127)

No doubt, the loss of a significant figure is likely to induce significant changes in the mourner's self that should be addressed. Thus, as previously indicated, the way the mourner perceives himself could be vastly affected by the loss. His sense of self-identity, self-worth, and self-cohesion could be undermined and give rise to feelings of vulnerability, and his value system could also undergo a significant change following the loss. However, as noted, it seems that the subjective experience of loss of a significant figure and its meaning for the bereaved have not been given due attention. The mental pain over the loss, the void left by the departed loved one that no substitute can fill, the feelings of empathy, identification, love, longing, guilt, anger, and other complex emotions about the deceased that are not necessarily directly related to changes in the mourner's self are no less relevant to the mourning process and likewise deserve consideration. The following case illustrates my point.

D., a patient of mine, lost her father at the age of 25 when he drowned at sea, rushing to the rescue of a child at risk. She described her father as a strong figure, a pillar of support in every respect (inter alia, financially), an attentive parent whose advice she had always sought. Her parents divorced when she was a little child. Her mother was kindhearted, but emotionally unstable, highly anxious, childish, behaviorally unexpected, and thus unreliable. Her relationship with her mother was characterized by role reversal, whereby as a parentified child, she felt deeply concerned about her mother and used to provide her with emotional and other required support. Her elder brother, who was already married with three children at the time, was a reserved and emotionally detached person, burdened by economic difficulties and health problems of one of his children and therefore unable to offer his sister emotional support. Upon the tragic loss of her father, D. felt that the ground slipped under her feet. Along with her agony over the loss, she felt exposed, vulnerable, and forced to struggle for survival. Her self-perception changed overnight. She was not used to feeling weak, incompetent, and ineffectual, feelings that gave rise to guilt and self-hate. Furthermore, she felt an outsider in her close social circle and envied her friends who could go on leading a normal life, untouched by trauma, which made her wonder whether she still had a common ground with them and if their past friendship could be truly maintained. With time, her interpersonal relationships underwent a change, in some respects, a change for the better (for instance, she felt less of a need to please her friends, whether old or new, and was more authentic and open in her social interactions). Other favorable changes in her life were evident later on, as manifested in her newly found interest in philanthropic projects and in her wish to get involved in initiatives on behalf of the community. She felt that these changes reflected a new perspective on life and on the priorities in her life. These were just some of the changes in the self, in part transient and in part enduring, undergone by D. following the death of her father. At the same time, her deep agony over the loss of her father and the unique emotional bond she had with him was striking. Far beyond the loss of the functions provided by him or the way she experienced herself following his death (i.e., her state of the self), his absence left a void that could not be filled. Three years after his death, she married a man who was eight years her senior and reminded her of her strong, supportive, and dependable father. Yet while, to a large extent, her spouse provided the functions previously provided by her father and, like her father, served as a significant selfobject for her, she still painfully missed her father and was occasionally overcome by intense longing for him. She shared with me her feelings of longing for her father, her memories of cherished moments with him, the acute pain over his absence that in a flash tore her heart ("as if the years haven't gone by and I've just been notified of his death"), her deep love for him, and even her feelings of guilt and anger (e.g., anger over his daring rescue feat that left her abandoned by him and his desertion of her mother in favor of another woman, who turned out to be cunning, manipulative, and abusive toward her and her brother). She often held imaginal dialogues with her father, asking for his opinion on various issues or seeking his protection from above. Thus, through the years, she maintained an enduring emotional bond and an ongoing dialogue with her departed father, even while another figure, her spouse, fulfilled the same functions previously fulfilled by her father for her.

Notably, Kernberg (2010), whose approach was essentially traditional, changed his position on the mourning process following the death of his wife, Paulina. Sharing his painful personal experience and its impact on his subsequent shift of position regarding normal mourning, Kernberg acknowledged that in line with the traditional psychoanalytic view, he used to see the mourner's continuing bond with the deceased as pathological and attributed his patients' failure to carry the mourning process to completion through ultimate emotional detachment from the departed dear one to feelings of guilt about or aggression toward the lost one. However, as he candidly admitted, his own personal experience and informal study of the experience of acquaintances who, like him, lost a dear life partner led him to the conclusion that the emotional bond with the deceased continued throughout life in various forms. Thus, even after long years, deep sadness and intense pain over the loss were still poignantly felt. The word *pain* recurrently used by Kernberg with reference to the mourning process reflects his intense subjective experience, which veiled the objective scientific perspective characteristic of his other writings. As Kernberg (2010) observed in this context:

> I propose that this objective absence in the presence of an intense subjective experience of the permanent relation between self and the lost other is at the center of the painful experience of loss and the compensatory processes this situation engenders.
>
> (p. 610)

While highlighting the natural phenomenon of continuing bond in a normal mourning process, Kernberg discussed, and duly so, the changes induced in the mourner's self by the loss of a dear one (or, as conceptualized by Kernberg, the significant structural changes in the ego, the superego, and the internalized representations of self and object), the way the mourner saw himself and the other following the loss, and the way in which the mourner's value systems and aspirations changed due to the loss in line with the internalized value systems of the lost one.

Apart from any other aspect of the mourning process (specifically the changes in the mourner's self), the focus on the painful separation from an irreplaceable, unique loved one, seen as a complex and enduring experience that is never carried to completion, reflects an awareness of the fundamental significance and unique nature of the relationship with a significant other – and hence of the emotional dependence on a specific significant other, which the narcissist would rather deny. The shift of psychoanalytic position on this issue, that is, its recognition of the mourner's lifelong emotional bond with the deceased (Gaines, 1997; Hagman, 2016; Kernberg, 2010; Sussillo, 2005), is reflected not only in the psychoanalytic literature but also in the wider theoretical and empirical literature that draws on numerous studies and extensive clinical experience (Cassidy & Shaver, 1999/2016; Neimeyer, 2016; Rubin, 1999). This mini-theory shift in psychoanalysis on the issue of bereavement and mourning was aptly referred to by Slochower (2011) as follows, "It is time for us to reject once and for all the psychoanalytic idealization of renunciation and separation, to embrace our (conflicted) desire and capacity for connection" (p. 180).

Indeed, maintaining a mental connection with the deceased is not only natural and normal but also conducive to the mourner's adaptation to life following the loss, as shown by various studies (reviewed by Sussillo, 2005). In line with the shift of position of psychoanalytic theory, the psychoanalytic approach to grief therapy has also been modified. Rather than encouraging complete emotional detachment from the departed dear one, current clinical practices aim to help the bereaved patient maintain an enduring bond with the deceased, even after working through mourning has supposedly been accomplished according to the traditional approach. This may be achieved by encouraging the bereaved to share his thoughts and feelings about the departed loved one and the void left by him, to hold imaginal dialogues with the lost one, or even talk to him as if he were present in the consulting room and thus experience his continued presence (Fraley & Shaver, 2016; Sussillo, 2005). It is a familiar psychotherapeutic technique applied in other contexts as well (Neimeyer, 2012; Neimeyer, 2016). It may be questioned, though, whether a continuing bond with the deceased is normal and conducive to adaptability in all cases and when it should be seen as reflecting a pathological mourning process. A pathological mourning process could be characterized by denial of the loss of the loved one and inability to accept the separation and carry on with normal life. The issue is too complex for extended discussion in this context. It appears, however, that paradoxically, the dialectic of a continuing bond with the deceased (*holding on*) and acceptance of the separation from the lost loved one (*letting go*) is indicative of a normal mourning process (Gaines, 1997; Sussillo, 2005). The separation from the deceased and return to involvement in all aspects of life is a gradual process that depends on the nature and circumstances of the loss as well as on the personality of the mourner. Carrying on with life in the deepest sense means finding a new meaning in life, re-engaging in former relationships or establishing new ones, experiencing positive emotions, restoring vitality, resuming normal functioning, and so on. The other aspect of the dialectical response to loss concerns, as noted, the enduring emotional bond with the deceased, including the whole gamut of thoughts and emotions stirred by this bond, the sorrow and pain over the loss, the memories of the deceased and the relationship with him, the attempt to cope with the void left by him, anger about him, unresolved issues that have to be settled, imaginal dialogues with the deceased, and more. The twofold response to loss discussed by Gaines and Sussillo corresponds to the two-track model of bereavement suggested by Rubin (1999), whereby the mourning process is "conceptualized along two distinct but interactive axes" (p. 681). One of the axes or tracks has to do with the return to normal life, including functioning in daily routine, engagement in interpersonal relationships, the presence or absence of various symptoms (e.g., anxiety, depression, somatic symptoms), self-perception, and the like. The other axis or track is focused on the mourner's continuing bond with the deceased and the nature of this bond. It is concerned with issues such as the extent to which the mourner is preoccupied with thoughts about the deceased; the mourner's imaginal relationship with the deceased and the changes in the relationship, if any, over the years; the emotions stirred in this context, whether positive or negative; and so forth. A normal mourning process would thus involve changes along both interactional tracks. The continuing bond with the deceased is, then, quite natural and, furthermore, has a highly significant role in the mourner's response to the loss – this, as long as it does not interfere with the mourner's ability to carry on with his life and engage emotionally with others, "balancing attachments to the living and the deceased" (p. 681). The following case illustrates a pathological response to loss.

H., a 30-year-old patient of mine who lost her brother in a car accident when she was 23, sought psychotherapy primarily due to tensions in her couple relationship over her doubts about having children. While her partner to life was all for it, H. felt an inexplicable resistance to the idea. She was also against having a formal marriage, which her partner did not really mind. They had been together for nine years at the time and living in a rented apartment. After some time in psychotherapy, it became clear that what stopped H. from moving on with her life and starting a family was guilt over the fact that her tragically lost brother would never experience parenthood or any other aspect of life as a mature adult. Thus, unconsciously, she did whatever she could to live her life as if time stood still, the way it was when her brother was still alive, denying her significantly changed life reality. She used to talk about him in an apparently casual manner, recalling moments of fun they had enjoyed together, and organized sing-along evenings featuring his favorite music. However, she did not leave room for the expression of her sadness and pain over the loss or her longing for her brother. Her family members and the friends of her brother knew that she did not want them to show their sympathy with her in her sorrow as it would only provoke anger and disaffection on her part. It appears, then, that H. was stopped in her tracks, as it were, upon the death of her brother, unable to accept the loss, cope with her feelings of guilt over the loss, and carry on with her life. In contrast, a healthy mourning process enables a continuing bond with the departed loved one, leaving room for a range of emotions and thoughts about the deceased, while facilitating a gradual return to life, the finding of meaning in life, and the creation of an emotional space for living life in full. In the case of H., eventually, with the progression of therapy, she came to accept the loss and, inter alia, realized that after all, she wished to have a child with her life partner.

Other non-narcissistic aspects

Other aspects of the discourse on the issue of mourning, although less focal, also reflect the reduction of the narcissistic bias in psychoanalytic theory.

Greater theoretical focus on normal mourning

Acknowledgment of the loss of a dear one, in general, and of the enduring feelings of pain and emptiness over the loss, in particular, reflects a basically non-narcissistic position. It necessarily entails recognition of our emotional dependence on the other and, furthermore, confronts us with the fundamental helplessness of human existence, with our limitations as humans, and with the transience of our existence. Most people tend to ignore the inevitable finality of life – theirs and that of their dear ones. Narcissists, more than others, are likely to outrightly deny their mortality. A corresponding narcissistic bias may be found in the traditional psychoanalytic literature on bereavement and mourning, which is primarily concerned with pathological mourning as reflected in clinical depression rather than with normal mourning (Kernberg, 2010). The discussion of bereavement and mourning from the pathological point of view supports the denial of that most basic aspect of human existence. Contemporary psychoanalytic literature, on the other hand, deals extensively with normal rather than with pathological mourning processes (Hagman, 2016; Kernberg, 2010) – a shift of focus that further reflects its toned-down narcissistic bias.

Description of the relationship with the deceased in positive, emotive, human terms

The mourning process is described in traditional psychoanalytic theory as a universal, mechanistic process that essentially involves the withdrawal of the libido from the deceased and its displacement to another one. However, such a description plays down the human experience of close interpersonal relationships, that is, the fundamental emotional bond between human beings. Conversely, contemporary psychoanalytic theory highlights the unique subjective experience of mourning and its ever-changing and, at the same time, enduring significance for the bereaved throughout life (Hagman, 2016). Furthermore, it deals extensively with the mourner's positive emotions about the deceased, whereas traditional psychoanalysis focused on the mourner's negative feelings of guilt about and aggression toward the deceased. Illustrative of the latter is Winnicott's view on loss and grief processes, as presented in his discussion of the psychology of separation (1984/1990)[4]:

> The mechanism of mourning is complex and includes the following: an individual subjected to loss of an object introjects the object and the object is subjected to hate within the ego. Clinically there is a variable deadness of the introjected object according to whether at one particular moment this object is more hated or more loved.
>
> (p. 114)

The mourner's feelings of hate, hostility, guilt, and ambivalence are highlighted elsewhere in Winnicott's writings and discussed in this context by other theorists as well (e.g., Kernberg, 2010). Undoubtedly, negative and ambivalent feelings are an inseparable part of any interpersonal relationship, including the mourner's ongoing relationship with a departed dear one. However, no less significant are the mourner's love for the lost one, his grief over the void left by the departed loved one, the beneficial role of the loved one in the mourner's life, and so on. Indeed, as noted, over the years, the focus has shifted toward a more positively toned portrayal of the subjective experience of mourning.

Discussion of mourning in the context of a matrix of interpersonal relationships

While the focus of traditional psychoanalytic theory was on mourning as an isolated intrapsychic process that concerned the mourner alone, the role of the other in mourning has recently been given special attention in the psychoanalytic discourse. The significance of a supportive surrounding for the mourner and its essential part in facilitating a normal mourning process by allowing a space for sharing, showing sympathy, offering emotional containment, providing selfobject functions, and so on are highlighted in contemporary psychoanalytic literature (Hagman, 1993; Hagman, 1996; Shane & Shane, 1990; Slochower, 2011).

Discussion of diverse types of losses

Psychoanalysis traditionally focused on the parent-infant relationship while failing to duly address the complexity of close relationships between adults, for instance, couple relationships (Kernberg, 2010), or relationships between siblings or close friends. Thus, the theories of Freud, Winnicott, and Kohut, which focus on the individual self, do not tell us much about mature, emotionally intimate interpersonal relationships. More recently, the psychoanalytic discussion of separation and loss has been expanded to include not only the impact of parental loss on the child but also other diverse types of losses. This shift of focus reflects a growing awareness of the significance of an enduring emotional bond between human beings in general, beyond the child-parent attachment relationship, as essential to the organization of the human psyche throughout life.

Notes

1 As noted, for the sake of brevity, the relational intersubjective school is referred to herein as the intersubjective school.
2 As openly expressed in his letters to Max Eitingon and Ludwig Binswanger, cited in Chapter 4.
3 This, in contrast to the traditional view of a normal mourning process as involving complete emotional detachment from the deceased.
4 Winnicott's view on the issue is discussed at more length in Chapter 4.

References

Beebe, B., & Lachmann, F. M. (2002). *Infant research and adult treatment: Co-constructing interactions*. The Analytic Press/Taylor & Francis Group.

Blatt, S. J. (2008). *Polarities of experience: Relatedness and self-definition in personality development, psychopathology, and the therapeutic process*. American Psychological Association.

Cassidy, J., & Shaver, P. R. (Eds.). (2016). *Handbook of attachment: Theory, research, and clinical applications*. (3rd ed.). Guilford Press. https://read.amazon.com/?asin=B01F9KHK4Y&ref_=kwl_kr_iv_rec_1 (Original work published 1999)

Deutsch, H. (1937). Absence of grief. *The Psychoanalytic Quarterly*, 6, 12–22.

Diamond, D. (2004). Attachment disorganization: The reunion of attachment theory and psychoanalysis. *Psychoanalytic Psychology, 21*(2), 276–299. https://doi.org/10.1037/0736-9735.21.2.276

Fonagy, P. (2018). *Attachment theory and psychoanalysis*. Routledge. (Original work published 2001)

Fraley, R. C., & Shaver, P. R. (2016). Attachment, loss, and grief: Bowlby's views, new developments, and current controversies. In J. Cassidy & P. R. Shaver (Eds.), *Handbook of attachment: Theory, research, and clinical applications* (3rd ed., pp. 40–62). Guilford Press. https://read.amazon.com/?asin=B01F9KHK4Y&ref_=kwl_kr_iv_rec_1

Freud, S. (1917). *Mourning and Melancholia* (J. Strachey, Ed. & Trans., in collaboration with Anna Freud, Standard Edition, Vol. 14, pp. 243–258). The Hogarth Press and the Institute of Psychoanalysis.

Freud, S. (1923). *The ego and the id and other works* (J. Strachey, Trans., Standard Edition, Vol. 19). The Hogarth Press and the Institute of Psychoanalysis.

Gaines, R. (1997). Detachment and continuity: The two tasks of mourning. *Contemporary Psychoanalysis, 33*(4), 549–571. https://doi.org/10.1080/00107530.1997.10747005

Hagman, G. (1993). The psychoanalytic understanding and treatment of double parent loss. In G. Hagman (Ed.), *New models of bereavement theory and treatment: New mourning* (pp. 39–54). Routledge.

Hagman, G. (1995). Self experience in mourning. In G. Hagman (Ed.), *New models of bereavement theory and treatment: New mourning* (pp. 115–129). Routledge.

Hagman, G. (1996). The role of the other in mourning. In G. Hagman (Ed.), *New models of bereavement theory and treatment: New mourning* (pp. 85–102). Routledge.

Hagman, G. (Ed.). (2016). *New models of bereavement theory and treatment: New mourning*. Routledge.

Harlem, A. (2009). Thinking through others: Cultural psychology and the psychoanalytic treatment of immigrants. *Psychoanalysis, Culture & Society, 14*(3), 273–288. https://doi.org/10.1057/pcs.2009.12

Kernberg, O. F. (2010). Some observations on the process of mourning. *The International Journal of Psychoanalysis, 91*(3), 601–619. https://doi.org/10.1111/j.1745-8315.2010.00286.x

Kohut, H. (1977). *The restoration of the self*. International Universities Press.

Kohut, H. (2011). *The search for the self: Selected writings of Heinz Kohut: 1978–1981. Vol. 4*. (P. H. Ornstein, Ed.). Karnac Books. https://read.amazon.com/?asin=B00582LHI4&ref_=kwl_kr_iv_rec_5 (Original work published 1991)

Magid, B., Fosshage, J., & Shane, E. (2021): The emerging paradigm of relational self psychology: An historical perspective. *Psychoanalysis, Self and Context, 16*(1), 1–23. https://doi.org/10.1080/24720038.2020.1856111

Mitchell, S. A. (2023). *Relationality: From attachment to intersubjectivity*. Routledge. https://read.amazon.com/?asin=B0B92S5PVW&ref_=kwl_kr_iv_rec_3 (Original work published 2000)

Neimeyer, R. A. (2012). Chair work. In R. A. Neimeyer (Ed.), *Techniques of grief therapy: Creative practices for counseling the bereaved* (pp. 266–273). Routledge/Taylor & Francis Group.

Neimeyer, R. A. (2016). Introduction. In G. Hagman (Ed.), *New models of bereavement theory and treatment: New mourning* (pp. xxiii–xxxix). Routledge.

Palombo, J. (1982). The psychology of the self and the termination of treatment. *Clinical Social Work Journal, 10*(1), 15–27.

Rubin, S. S. (1999). The two-track model of bereavement: Overview, retrospect, and prospect. *Death Studies, 23*(8), 681–714. https://doi.org/10.1080/074811899200731

Shane, E., & Shane, M. (1990). Object loss and selfobject loss: A contribution to understanding mourning and the failure to mourn. In G. Hagman (Ed.), *New models of bereavement theory and treatment: New mourning* (pp. 24–38). Routledge.

Shelby, R. D. (1994). Mourning theory reconsidered. In G. Hagman (Ed.), *New models of bereavement theory and treatment: New mourning* (pp. 66–84). Routledge.

Slochower, J. (2011). Out of the analytic shadow: On the dynamics of commemorative ritual. In G. Hagman (Ed.), *New models of bereavement theory and treatment: New mourning* (pp. 167–184). Routledge.

Sussillo, M.V. (2005). Beyond the grave – Adolescent parental loss: Letting go and holding on. *Psychoanalytic Dialogues, 15*(4), 499–527. https://doi.org/10.1080/10481881509348846

Togashi, K., & Kottler, A. (2021). From a cohesive self to a relational being: The evolution of the psychology of the self to the psychology of being human. *Psychoanalytic Inquiry, 41*(3), 187–198.

Winnicott, D. W. (1990). *Deprivation and delinquency* (C. Winnicott, R. Shepherd, & M. Davis, Eds.). Routledge. (Original work published 1984)

8 Reflections on the current status of psychoanalysis as a therapeutic method

Are we witness to the sinking of the *Titanic*?

It goes without saying that throughout its history psychoanalysis has played a key role in our understanding of deep-seated, complex mental processes. Yet while the body of theoretical psychoanalytic knowledge offers invaluable insights, the current relevance of psychoanalysis as an effective or desirable therapeutic method seems to be in doubt, as discussed hereinafter. To consider the effectiveness and suitability of psychoanalysis as a therapeutic method, we have first to answer the question, what is psychoanalysis? However, there is no consensus about the criteria that distinguish psychoanalysis as a therapeutic method. And given the diversity of psychoanalytic schools and their widely divergent views on key issues, such as the primary goals of psychoanalytic treatment, the type of the therapeutic setting, and the analyst's role in the therapeutic encounter, there is no simple, clear-cut answer to the question. Thus, for instance, one may wonder whether the classical psychoanalytic approach of Freud, Klein, and their present-day successors (e.g., Blass, 2011; Kernberg, 2018), which sees the Oedipal complex, aggressiveness, sexuality, and the related mental conflicts as governing the human psyche, can be reconciled with the spiritually sensitive psychoanalysis advocated by Eigen (2001), Lev (2015), and Kulka (2008), among others, which focuses on morality, compassion, and generosity, drawing on various traditions and influences, notably Buddhism. Likewise, one may question whether there can be a common ground between psychoanalysts who believe that the analyst should maintain a neutral position in the analytic dialogue (e.g., Kernberg, 2021; Ogden, 1996) and psychotherapists who hold that the analyst should highlight his subjective presence in the therapeutic encounter, at times taking it too far, to the point of excessive self-disclosure (Davies, 1994; Renik, 1993, 2006). Equally controversial are questions such as, is it knowledge that the patient is in need of and awareness of his mental world, or is it rather a corrective experience in the space of the therapeutic relationship, where his authentic self can be expressed and his inhibited creativity flourish? Even the most basic issue of whether psychoanalysis can offer universal truths is subject to dispute. Relational and intersubjective theorists question the very

DOI: 10.4324/9781003538295-8

existence of universally applicable absolute truths, while others believe that certain truths can and should be considered fundamental tenets.[1] It seems as if psychoanalysis has become a subjective object, to use Winnicott's terminology, interpreted by each school in light of its views and beliefs and actually, restructured at will. Notwithstanding the differences and, in some cases, apparently unbridgeable gap between the various approaches, Aron and Starr (2013) sought to find a common ground rather than dwell on the disagreements. Their quest to bring together divergent perspectives seems to be driven by their concern about the ongoing decline of psychoanalysis, the once dominant therapeutic method:

> Psychoanalysis has clearly suffered from decline in status and demand, fewer applicants to our institutes, fewer patients, greater competition, less reimbursement, higher demands for empirical research, less support in departments of psychology, and almost none in psychiatry. Sales of psychoanalytic books are at an all-time record low.
>
> (p. 11)

Eisold (2005) pointed to the same downward trend, as reflected in the various surveys conducted by renowned bodies, including the International Psychoanalytic Association. Indeed, it seems that this continuing downward trend threatens the future of psychoanalysis as a therapeutic method (Kernberg, 2021).

Aron and Starr (2013) criticized the preoccupation with the dividing lines between the various psychoanalytic schools, the focus on the definition of psychoanalysis, and the disputes about trivialities, as they saw it, evoking the sinking *Titanic* metaphor to drive their point home:

> We have often felt that the bickering among psychoanalysts about what "counts" as psychoanalysis, what theory, how many times per week, whether or not the couch is used, what school of thought is included or excluded, is nothing more than rearranging the chairs on the Titanic as the ship is sinking.
>
> (p. 8)

Looking for a common denominator between the various psychoanalytic schools, Aron and Starr cited the empirically based criteria[2] suggested by Shedler (2010) for characterizing analytic therapies as distinct from nonanalytic therapies, as presented next in short form:

1. **Analytic therapists focus on affect and the expression of emotions**
   "The therapist helps the patient describe and put words to feelings, including contradictory feelings, feelings that are troubling or threatening, and feelings that the patient may not initially be able to recognize or acknowledge" (Shedler, 2010, p. 99).

2. **Exploration of attempts to avoid distressing thoughts and feelings**
   He [Shedler] explains the psychodynamic therapist's focus on defense mechanisms, giving as illustrations avoidance, externalization, isolation of affect, and shifts in free association.
3. **Identification of recurring themes and patterns**
   The psychoanalytic therapist[3] explores themes and patterns, including those that the patient had not noticed or recognized previously.
4. **Discussion of past experience – a developmental focus**
   Exploring . . . early experiences and "the ways in which the past tends to 'live on' in the present" (p. 99). The goal is to help patients free themselves from the bonds of past experience.
5. **Focus on interpersonal relations**
   exploring the patient's patterns of interpersonal relations (both internal and external), attachment patterns, and object-relations.
6. **Focus on the therapy relationship**
   in the specific focus on the therapy relationship . . . we get to what is usually described as transference and countertransference. . . . He [Shedler] is careful to note that . . . the therapy relationship provides a unique opportunity to explore and rework these often unconscious patterns in vivo.
7. **Exploration of fantasy life**
   The psychoanalytic therapist uses a less structured approach than other therapists, encouraging "patients to speak freely about whatever is on their minds" (p. 100). Here Shedler is describing what is usually called free association.

(Aron & Starr, 2013, pp. 375–376)

In addition to these seven empirically based criteria, Shedler (2010) suggested a key criteria of his own, noting that beyond symptom remission or relief of distress, the goal of psychoanalytic-psychodynamic therapy was to "foster the positive presence of psychological capacities and resources" (p. 100).

The criteria suggested by Shedler provide a common ground, albeit rather general, for defining psychoanalytically oriented therapies as distinct from therapies offered by other schools. However, while no doubt of value, this distinction fails to define the difference between psychoanalysis and in-depth, dynamic psychotherapy, which although overlapping in certain significant respects, are essentially distinct. Seeking to distinguish between the two, Mitchell and Black (1995/2016) considered the characterization of psychoanalysis versus psychotherapy:

> Should shorter treatments, less frequent sessions, and face-to-face work still be considered psychoanalysis? Or should the term psychoanalysis be reserved for the traditional, formal analytic setting, and the term psychotherapy be used in relation to the wide range of modifications

> now being practiced? There has been a great deal of debate in the literature about how psychoanalysis, in contrast to psychotherapy, should be defined. Gill (1994) has argued that the formal, "extrinsic" criteria – three or four sessions a week, the couch, and so on – should themselves not be the basis for calling a treatment psychoanalytic; for Gill, what is definitive of psychoanalysis are the "intrinsic" criteria: the depth of the process and the systematic exploration of transference-countertransference issues. Some argue that a true analytic process of in-depth work with transference phenomena cannot happen with one or two sessions a week, or without the couch, or in treatments of short duration. Others (including Gill) argue that the deepest dynamic issues and transference-countertransference interactions can emerge in many different circumstances, if the analyst is willing to focus on and engage them. The debate goes on and will go on for some time.
>
> (pp. 251–252)

Given the aforesaid, the basic differences between psychoanalysis and psychotherapy regarding which there is a rather broad agreement are described next. A number of key issues pointing to the underlying narcissistic bias characteristic of psychoanalysis, as contrasted with psychoanalytically oriented psychotherapy, are discussed in this context. It should be noted that due to the diversity of psychoanalytic schools and their widely divergent views, the main distinguishing characteristics discussed here may not accurately represent some psychoanalytic approaches, although this should not detract from the picture as a whole.

The "extrinsic" criteria cited by Mitchell and Black (1995/2016) are highly significant in my mind and enable a good enough distinction between psychoanalysis and psychotherapy. It is widely agreed that a therapeutic setting of three to five sessions a week, usually conducted over many years, and the use of the analytic couch, on which the patient lies, out of direct eye contact with the analyst, who sits behind the couch, characterize psychoanalytic treatment. This therapeutic setting encourages the patient's regressivity, facilitates exploration of the patient's fantasy life, and occupies a large part of his life. In contrast, the therapeutic setting of psychotherapy is less demanding and less regressive. It typically involves one or occasionally two sessions a week, conducted with the analyst and patient sitting face-to-face, in direct eye contact, and it is usually of significantly shorter duration compared with psychoanalysis, lasting from a few months to a couple of years. Beyond the extrinsic criteria of the therapeutic setting, the position adopted by the analyst, his presence in the analytic discourse, the nature of the therapeutic interventions, and the therapy foci differ between psychoanalysis and psychotherapy. In psychoanalytic treatment, the analyst tends to stay more or less in the background and encourages the patient to engage in free association, focusing on the exploration of the patient's fantasy life. As part of the process, emphasis is placed on the transference-countertransference relationship, whereas the patient's past and present life reality and interpersonal relationships outside the consultation room are given less attention, as reflected in the clinical approach of Ogden (1996) and Kernberg (2021). Furthermore, the therapeutic goals of psychoanalysis are largely amorphous and general and concern the patient's personality as a whole. Thus, for instance, psychoanalytic treatment aims at enriching the self, improving the capacity to maintain intersubjective relationships, fostering meaning making, enhancing awareness of the self, promoting contact with the fundamental truths of human existence, and more.[4] On the other hand, in psychotherapy, the analyst assumes a relatively active role, managing the analytic discourse as a less associative dialogue (McWilliams, 2011), while leaving room for addressing the patient's life reality and setting more concrete and focused therapeutic goals. At the same time, in-depth psychotherapy, the way I see it, looks at the wider picture of the patient's personality, including his mental resources and difficulties, and as noted by Shedler (2010), rather than dealing merely with specific symptoms, seeks to lead to an overall change in the patient's life.

Indeed, the psychoanalyst generally does not, and as argued by Orange (2011), should not see himself as an expert whose mission is to cure his patients but rather as a facilitating agent, as it were, whose presence and interventions set in motion a comprehensive, in-depth development process. Already Winnicott (1989/2018) observed in the same spirit:

> Psycho-analysis does not cure, though it is true that a patient may make use of psycho-analysis, and may achieve with adjunctive process a degree of integration and socialization and self-discovery which he would not or could not have achieved without it.
>
> (p. 216)

Bion took it even further, noting that the passion to cure the patient obstructed the therapeutic process. According to Bion, a cure, if achieved, is a secondary by-product of psychoanalysis. To get to the deepest levels of the patient's unconscious mind, the analyst has to meet his patient with no desire to cure him and with no memory of past sessions or of the mental content that emerged during those sessions. It is this intuitive, nonsensuous approach to the exploration of psychic reality that enables us to come into contact with the ultimate truths of human existence, the unknowable ultimate reality – the domain of O, as Bion termed it (Symington & Symington, 1996).

The psychoanalytic culture of not knowing, which has its roots in the past,[5] has gained momentum in recent years with the emergence of intersubjectivity theory, which, drawing on postmodern ideas, questions the certainty and universality of objective knowledge and truth. Thus, the analyst is not required to know what is going on in the mental world of the patient, describe the patient's intrapsychic dynamics, or put his finger on the problem. Indeed, the analyst is urged to acknowledge his uncertainty, rely on his subjective experience, and thereby open up to processes of significance to the analytic dyad in the therapeutic encounter. Referring to the glorification of the position of not knowing in the psychoanalytic culture, Mitchell (1993) observed:

> Whereas earlier generations of psychoanalysts prided themselves on knowing and being brave enough to know, the current generation of psychoanalytic authors tends increasingly to stress the value of not knowing and the courage that requires. A growing chorus of voices from quite different psychoanalytic traditions stresses the enormous complexity and fundamental ambiguity of experience.
>
> (p. 42)

As further noted by Mitchell, the analyst's position of not knowing is actually seen as a measure of excellence:

> Other authors and practitioners who still believe they know things are often portrayed as fainthearted worshipers of illusions. In a reversal of traditional psychoanalytic machismo, it now sometimes appears that the capacity to contain the dread of not knowing is a measure of analytic virtue; the fewer convictions, the better and the braver!
>
> (p. 43)

It can be said, then, that in general, psychoanalysis focuses on comprehensive personality development rather than on the treatment of specific symptoms or relief of distress, while it tends to see the analyst as less of an expert who has a clear picture of his patient's mental state.[6] The broadly defined, amorphous therapeutic goals of psychoanalysis, which are aimed at setting in motion an overall development process and enhancing the patient's personality as a whole, are no doubt important, but in many cases, they do not meet the patient's needs and expectations for solution to a specific problem or change in a specific area of his life. Most of those who seek mental therapy, whatever the type of therapy, look up to the therapist, hoping for a cure for their distress, and when they do not find an adequate response, they look for another kind of therapy. At present, they can choose from an array of alternative options that are available for shorter-term, less costly, and less burdensome therapy, whether psychoanalytically oriented in-depth psychotherapy or symptom-focused treatments such as cognitive behavioral therapy (CBT) or eye movement desensitization and reprocessing (EMDR) therapy. Even Renik (2006), who is firmly rooted in the psychoanalytic establishment, is critical of psychoanalysis as a therapeutic method, noting its failure to attend to the patient's specific needs and deliver practical solutions to his specific problems. Indeed, as noted, psychoanalysis as a therapeutic method encourages engagement in an alternative, regressive, self-contained reality while failing to take due account of the patient's true life reality and special needs and concerns for which he seeks relief and is thus narcissistically biased. In contrast, the proposed non-narcissistic in-depth psychotherapy takes note of and responds to the patient's specific needs while considering the broad picture of his personality and life reality.

It appears that psychoanalysis as a therapeutic method is, in fact, in danger of extinction, first and foremost due to its narcissistic position, and we may thus wonder whether it is the sinking of the *Titanic* that we are witness to. It should be noted, though, that while psychoanalysis is increasingly less relevant as a therapeutic method, there is no question about the relevance of psychoanalysis as a theory of the human mind. The rich body of psychoanalytic knowledge offers invaluable insights into human nature (McWilliams, 2020), which can be applied in various psychotherapeutic methods, in particular, non-narcissistically oriented psychotherapy that is based on psychoanalytic concepts and principles.

Non-narcissistically oriented psychotherapy

The discussion of narcissism and psychoanalysis in this book indicates what should be considered, in my opinion, a non-narcissistically biased theoretical position and how it should be applied in clinical practice. It is suggested that in-depth psychotherapy provides a non-narcissistic framework for treatment by responding to the patient's specific needs while considering the broad picture of his personality and life reality. As noted, the therapeutic setting characteristic of in-depth psychotherapy is less demanding in terms of both session frequency and therapy duration compared with psychoanalysis. It is also less regressive and more focused on achieving concrete therapeutic goals aimed at leading to change in one or more areas of the patient's life. The therapeutic approach as bearing on the analyst's position vis-à-vis the patient and on the nature of the analytic encounter is further discussed next.

Like Blatt (2008), I believe that the need for interpersonal relatedness as well as the need for the development of the self and the expression of the self are both fundamental, universal human needs. The development of the self, traditionally a prime goal of the therapeutic process, can be promoted by the analyst in various ways, whether by enhancing the patient's awareness of his mental world, by encouraging the patient's self-enrichment and strengthening his self-cohesiveness, by supporting the patient in coping with mental conflicts, or by bolstering his resilience in the face of adversity and crisis. Yet it is no less important that the patient be directly encouraged to engage in real-life interpersonal relationships (Wachtel, 2009). Rather than hoping for change in the dimension of relatedness merely by focusing on self-development, the analyst should directly focus on the patient's real-life relationships, inter alia, by gradually bringing him into contact with his innate, deep-rooted yearning for emotional intimacy, which he may deny due to his schizoid personality traits. Thus, for instance, I once told a patient of mine, "When you are talking about your colleague at work, my impression is that you wish to have a closer, more intimate relationship with her rather than just serving as the supportive friend at time of crisis, lending an ear following her breakup with her boyfriend. Would you like to share any thoughts or feelings you have about it?"

The analyst is required not only to be sensitive to the most subtle signs of the patient's wish for close interpersonal relationships but also to legitimize, as it were, the patient's wish for emotional intimacy and encourage him to take the risk and get involved in a close emotional relationship. The analyst's intervention in this respect may also be called for in the case of a pathological mourning process following the loss of a significant figure, which could get in the way of the patient's emotional involvement in other relationships. Another case that may necessitate direct intervention in the aspect of relatedness is that of a patient who avoids involvement in any kind of relationship, whether interpersonal, social, or communal, due to fear of rejection, a low self-esteem, and the like. Evidently, the two dimensions of self-definition and relatedness reciprocally impact, shape, and reinforce each other. However, the therapeutic focus should be on the weaker dimension to ensure a balanced outcome and hence significant improvement in the patient's well-being.

Equally important, to respond to the specific needs of the patient, the analyst has to discuss with him and accordingly set the goals for therapy. At the same time, while attentively listening to the patient's complaints and wishes, the analyst should get an in-depth, comprehensive picture of the patient so as to better understand him, his personality, and the source of his mental difficulties, of which the patient may be aware or unaware, and as needed, jointly redefine the therapeutic goals. It should be noted that the therapeutic goals thus defined are not meant to be practical in the narrow, superficial sense of the word or necessarily offer a direct response to a specific complaint of the patient. Rather, the analyst should take into consideration various aspects of the patient's personality that may account for his mental difficulties, including dominant personality traits, the level of personality organization, and any observable symptoms (Kernberg, 2021; Lingiardi et al., 2015; McWilliams, 2011) as well as formative life events and, based on a comprehensive personality assessment, enable an inclusive development process while, at the same time, providing suitable interventions adapted to the patient's specific needs. The therapeutic goals related to the patient's diagnosed difficulties and other aspects of his life and personality should be clearly communicated by the analyst along with the expected outcome of the therapeutic process as regards both the issues that the patient seeks to address in therapy and those that emerge during the process. Thus, to cite another case, a patient of mine who sought therapy due to depression was found to have difficulty with identifying his needs and wishes and authentically expressing his true self. While attending to his depression, the therapeutic process was aimed at raising his self-awareness and enhancing his ability to express and realize denied aspects of his life. That is, beyond dealing with a specific issue – in this case, the patient's depression, its underlying causes, and its relief – the therapeutic process presented the patient with an in-depth, comprehensive picture of his condition and launched a development process that impacted his quality of life in general.

As argued, it is the patient rather than the therapeutic relationship that should be at the center of attention. To be sure, the relationship between analyst and patient is highly significant for the patient in various respects, as reflected, inter alia, in the enactment of early childhood relationships and subsequent corrective experience through the transference relationship, where the analyst serves in the role of a beneficial parental figure. The mutually influential intersubjective relationship between analyst and patient is likewise noteworthy in this context, and the same is true for the use of here-and-now processes emerging in the therapeutic encounter to deal with various issues of relatedness, including the otherness of the other, represented by the therapist. However, significant as it may be, the focus on the therapeutic relationship in the analytic discourse to the virtual exclusion of outside reality (Wachtel, 2009) produces (as noted in Chapter 6) a malignant narcissistic glass bubble.

Last but not least, the analyst should adopt a flexible position vis-à-vis the patient, moving between an organizing, supportive, explanatory, guiding, and knowledgeable approach (allowing for slip-ups and further examination) that deals with objective reality, on the one hand, and a stance of open-mindedness that leaves room for the world of illusion and fantasy and the nebulous, associative, experiential, and regressive potential spaces, where both analyst and patient are groping their way in the unknowable darkness. Balancing between the two would enable the analyst to acknowledge objective reality and its impact on the patient while exploring the deep-seated inner world of the patient and thus, hand in hand with the patient, come into contact with unexpected truths and surprising revelations, going through enriching experiences that strengthen the self and its resources.

Notes

1 Freud's position on the issue, reflected in his statement (cited in Chapter 6), *I don't believe in relativity, I believe in absolute truths* (Rolnik, 2019), is noteworthy in this context.

2 Specifically, as noted by Aron and Starr (2013, p. 375), empirical studies identified by Blagys and Hilsenroth (2000) that compared manualized psychodynamic therapy with manualized cognitive behavioral therapy (CBT).

3 As noted by Aron and Starr (2013, p. 374), "He [Shedler] used the terms psychodynamic and psychoanalytic interchangeably, since his focus was on psychoanalytic therapy rather than on psychoanalysis proper."

4 Naturally, each psychoanalytic school has its own specific goals, based on its approach and beliefs.

5 For instance, Winnicott (1965) believed that "It is very important . . . that the analyst shall *not* know the answers except in so far as the patient gives the clues" (p. 50). Kohut (1984) advocated introspection and empathy rather than extrospection as the ultimate tool for accessing and understanding the patient's inner world. Bollas (1989/2018) maintained that to come into contact with the analysand's unconscious, the analyst has to assume no a priori knowledge.

6 There are exceptions, of course, e.g., the Kleinians as well as the Kernbergians, who believe that they have hold of the truth and see the analyst as a knowledgeable expert who seeks to unravel the objective truth about the patient.

References

Aron, L., & Starr, K. (2013). *A psychotherapy for the people: Toward a progressive psychoanalysis*. Routledge/Taylor & Francis Group.

Blass, R. B. (2011). On the immediacy of unconscious truth: Understanding Betty Joseph's 'here and now' through comparison with alternative views of it outside of and within Kleinian thinking. *The International Journal of Psychoanalysis, 92*(5), 1137–1157. https://doi.org/10.1111/j.1745-8315.2010.00361.x

Blatt, S. J. (2008). *Polarities of experience: Relatedness and self-definition in personality development, psychopathology, and the therapeutic process*. American Psychological Association.

Bollas, C. (2018). *Forces of destiny: Psychoanalysis and human idiom*. Routledge. https://doi.org/10.4324/9781315533414 (Original work published 1989)

Davies, J. M. (1994). Love in the afternoon: A relational reconsideration of desire and dread in the countertransference. *Psychoanalytic Dialogues, 4*(2), 153–170.

Eigen, M. (2001). *Ecstasy*. Wesleyan University Press.

Eisold, K. (2005). Psychoanalysis and psychotherapy: A long and troubled relationship. *The International Journal of Psychoanalysis, 86*(4), 1175–1195. https://doi.org/10.1516/8RMN-4EQF-LG1E-JG03

Kernberg, O. F. (2018). *Treatment of severe personality disorders: Resolution of aggression and recovery of eroticism*. American Psychiatric Association.

Kernberg, O. F. (2021). Extensions of psychoanalytic technique: The mutual influences of standard psychoanalysis and transference-focused psychotherapy. *Psychodynamic Psychiatry, 49*(4), 506–531.

Kohut, H. (1984). *How does analysis cure?* (A. Goldberg, Ed., with P. E. Stepansky). The University of Chicago Press. https://read.amazon.com/?asin=B015KJZF8M&ref_=kwl_kr_iv_rec_1

Kulka, R. (2008). From a discontented culture to a culture of compassion. In G. Shefler (Ed.), *Freud, culture and psychoanalysis: New readings of "civilization and its discontents"* (pp. 98–121). Dvir & Magnes. [Hebrew]

Lev, G. (2015). Morality, selflessness, transcendence: On treatment goals of a spiritually sensitive psychoanalysis. *Contemporary Psychoanalysis, 51*(3), 523–556.

Lingiardi, V., McWilliams, N., Bornstein, R. F., Gazzillo, F., & Gordon, R. M. (2015). *The psychodynamic diagnostic manual version 2 (PDM-2)*: Assessing patients for improved clinical practice and research. *Psychoanalytic Psychology, 32*(1), 94–115. https://doi.org/10.1037/a0038546

McWilliams, N. (2011). *Psychoanalytic diagnosis: Understanding personality structure in the clinical process* (2nd ed.). Guilford Press.

McWilliams, N. (2020). The future of psychoanalysis: Preserving Jeremy Safran's integrative vision. *Psychoanalytic Psychology, 37*(2), 98–107. https://doi.org/10.1037/pap0000275

Mitchell, S. A. (1993). *Hope and dread in psychoanalysis*. Basic Books.

Mitchell, S. A., & Black, M. J. (2016). *Freud and beyond: A history of modern psychoanalytic thought*. Basic Books. https://read.amazon.com/?asin=B06XBVPQGS&ref_=kwl_kr_iv_rec_1 (Original work published 1995)

Ogden, T. H. (1996). Reconsidering three aspects of psychoanalytic technique. *The International Journal of Psychoanalysis, 77*(5), 883–899.

Orange, D. M. (2011). *The suffering stranger: Hermeneutics for everyday clinical practice*. Routledge.

Renik, O. (1993). Analytic interaction: Conceptualizing technique in light of the analyst's irreducible subjectivity. *Psychoanalytic Quarterly, 62*(4), 553–571.
Renik, O. (2006). *Practical psychoanalysis for therapists and patients*. Other Press.
Rolnik, E. (2019). *Sigmund Freud – Letters*. Modan. [Hebrew]
Shedler, J. (2010). The efficacy of psychodynamic psychotherapy. *American Psychologist, 65*(2), 98–109.
Symington, J., & Symington, N. (1996). *The clinical thinking of Wilfred Bion*. Routledge.
Wachtel, P. L. (2009). Knowing oneself from the inside out, knowing oneself from the outside in – The "Inner" and "Outer" worlds and their link through action. *Psychoanalytic Psychology, 26*(2), 158–170. https://doi.org/10.1037/a0015502
Winnicott, D. W. (1965). *The maturational processes and the facilitating environment Studies in the theory of emotional development*. International Universities Press.
Winnicott, D. W. (2018). *Psycho-analytic explorations* (C. Winnicott, R. Shepherd, & M. Davis, Eds.). Routledge. (Original work published 1989)

Index

FSC
www.fsc.org
MIX
Papier | Fördert
gute Waldnutzung
FSC® C083411

Kolibri 360 GmbH
Ferdinand-Jühlke-Straße 7
99095 Erfurt, Deutschland
produktsicherheit@kolibri360.de